ONE Good Egg

Based On a True Story

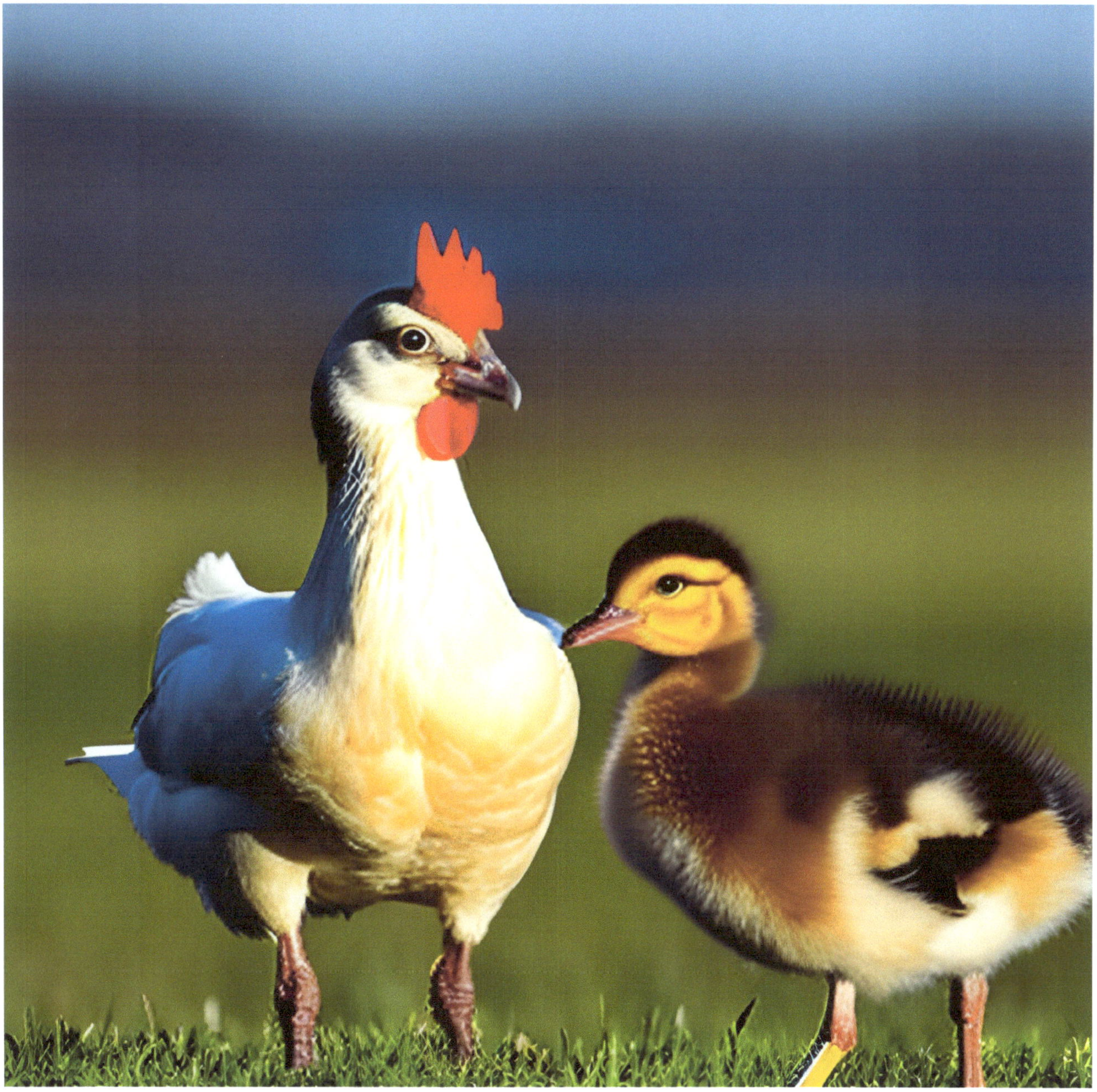

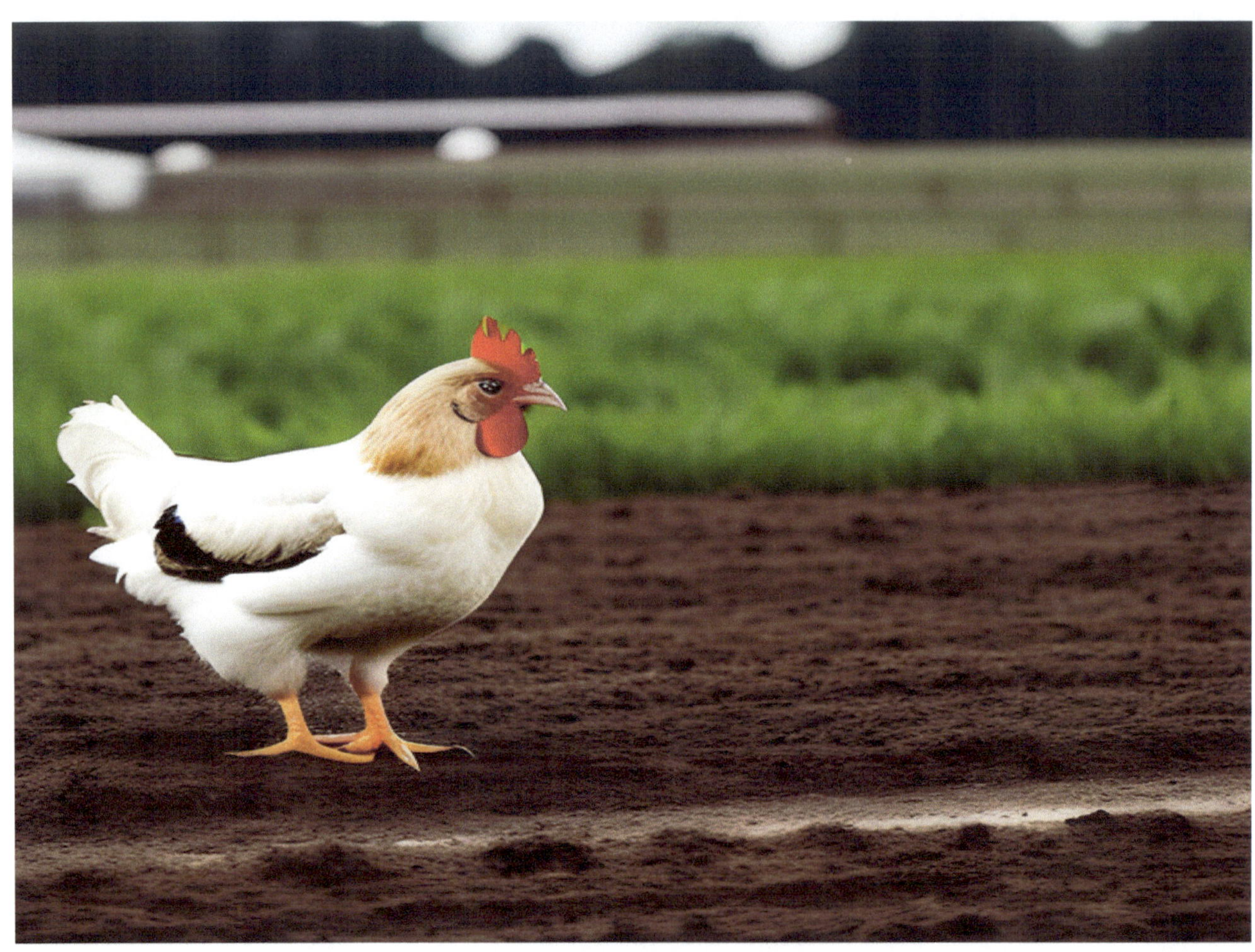

Once upon a time there was a chicken named Grace. Grace lived on a lovely farm in Florida.

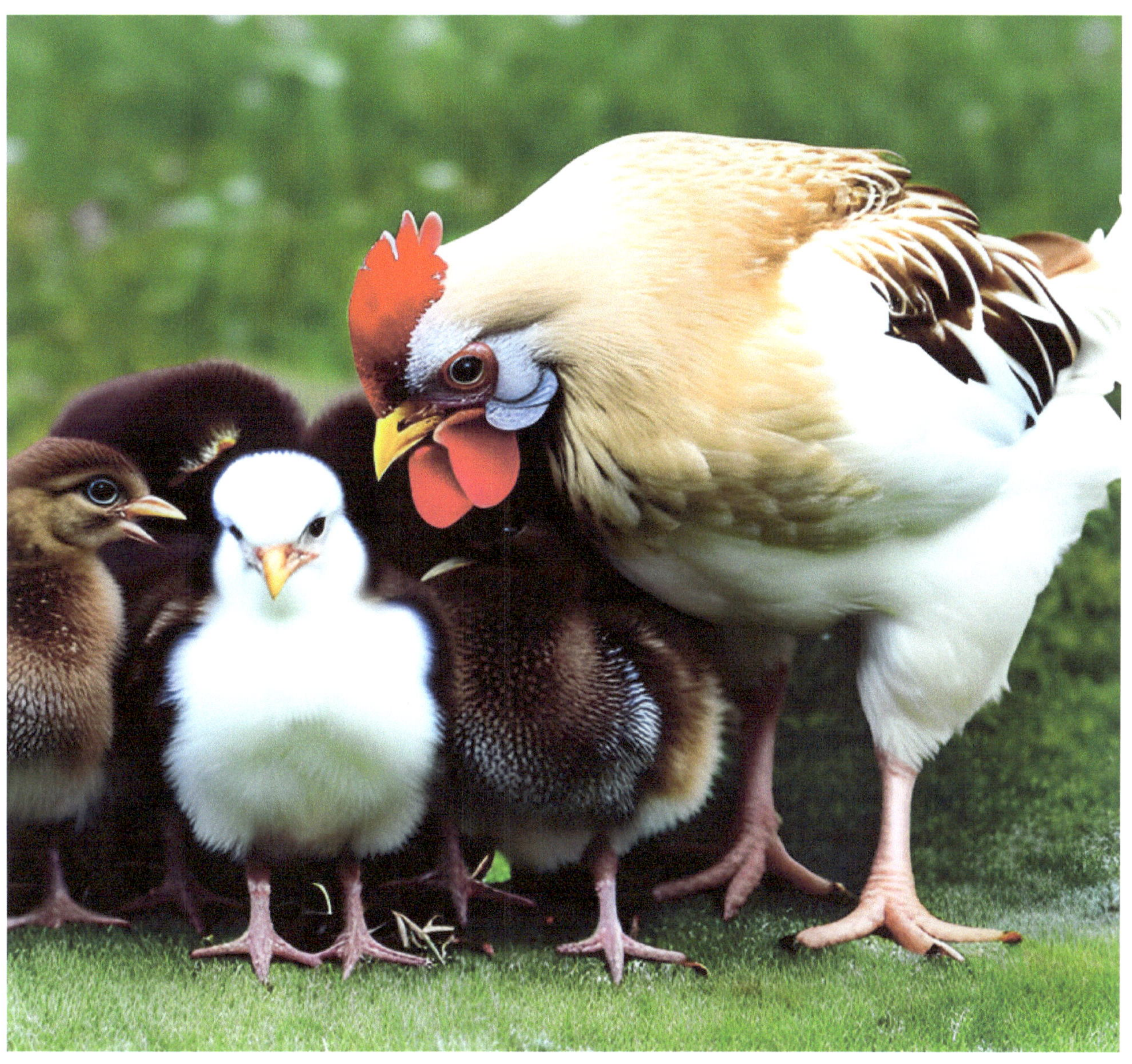

Grace was a happy chicken, but Grace had a dream of being a mom ever since she had been a chick.

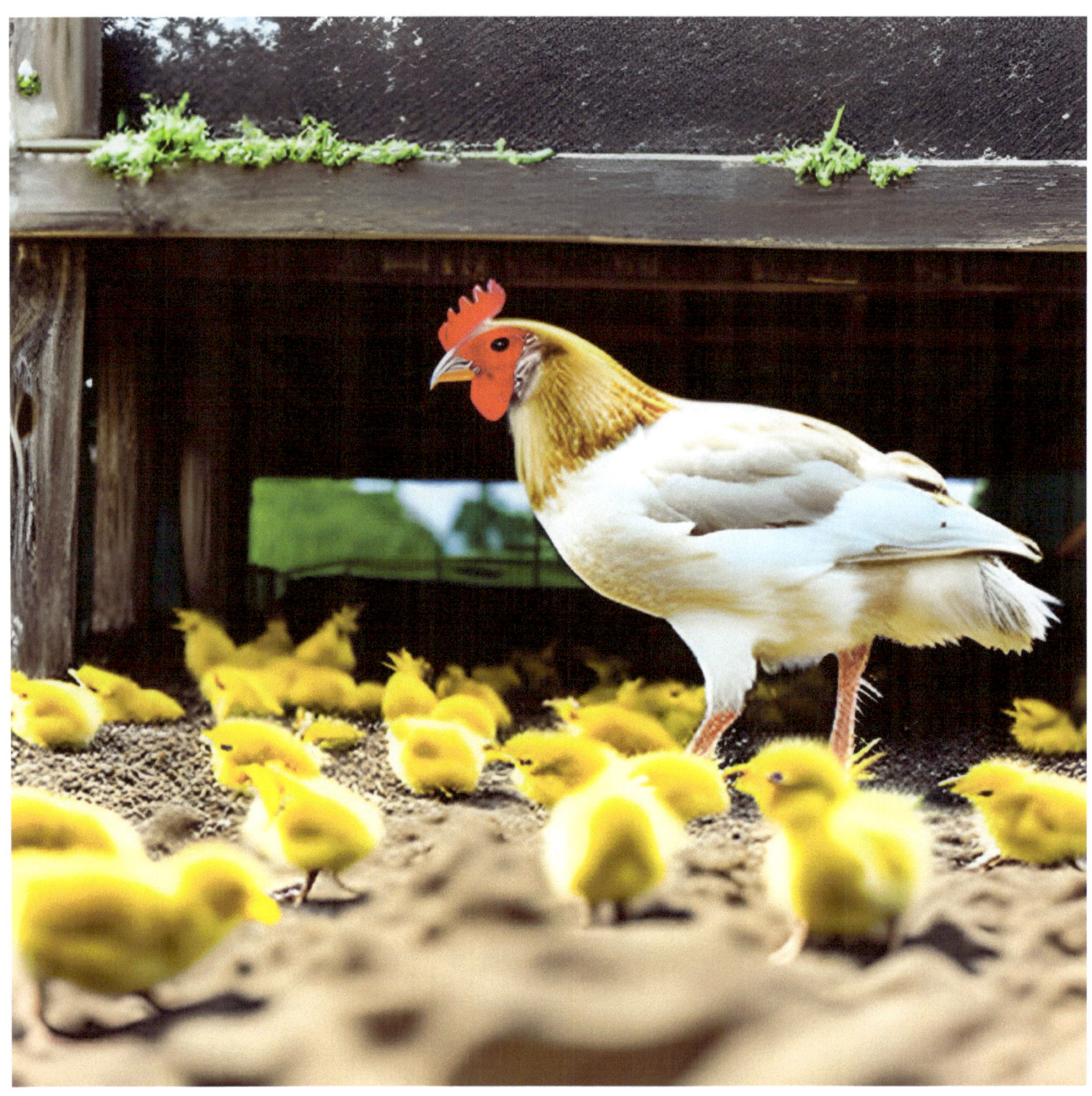

Grace loved watching the cute chicks play with their mothers on the farm.

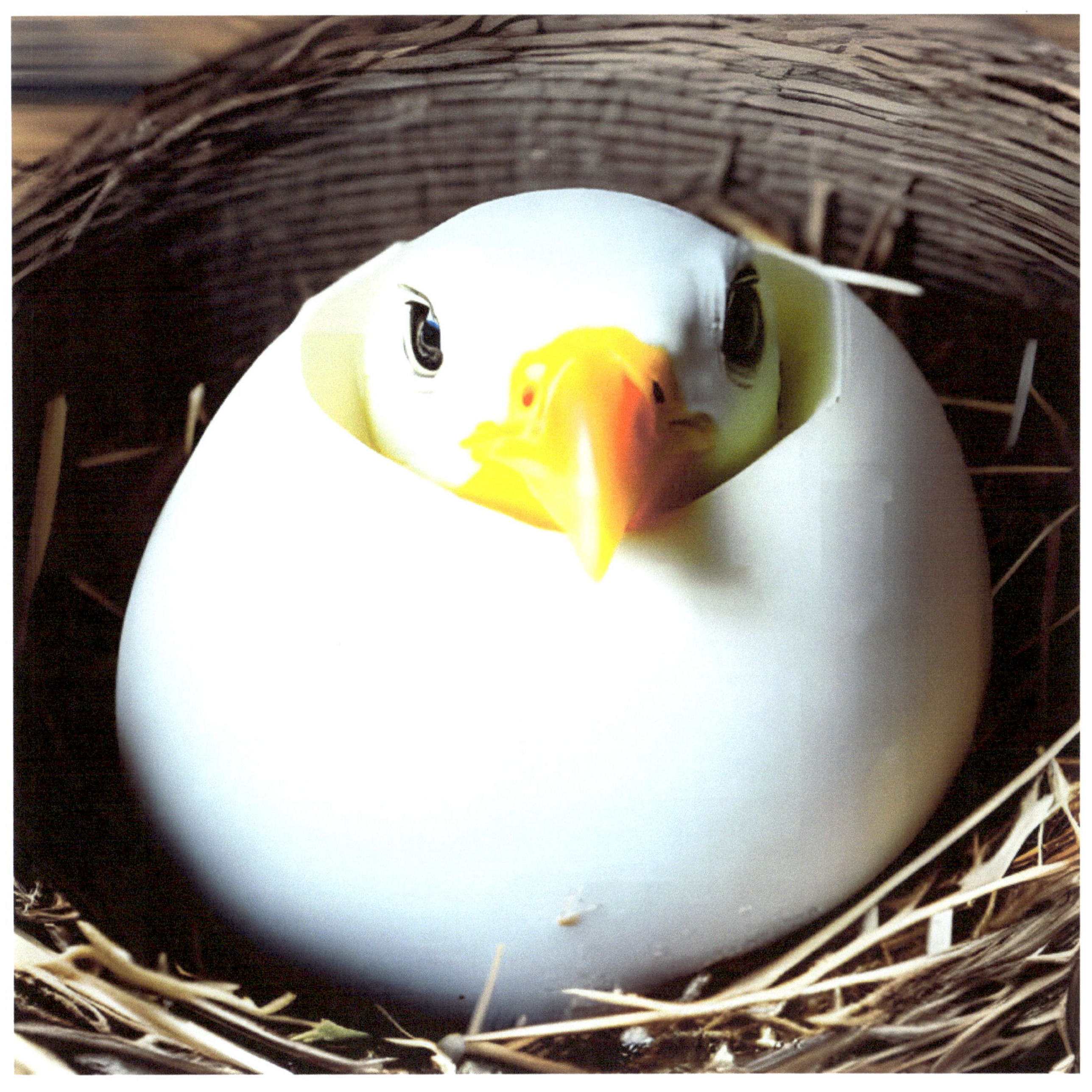

Grace also loved watching the cute chicks hatch under their mothers and knew one day her egg would hatch too.

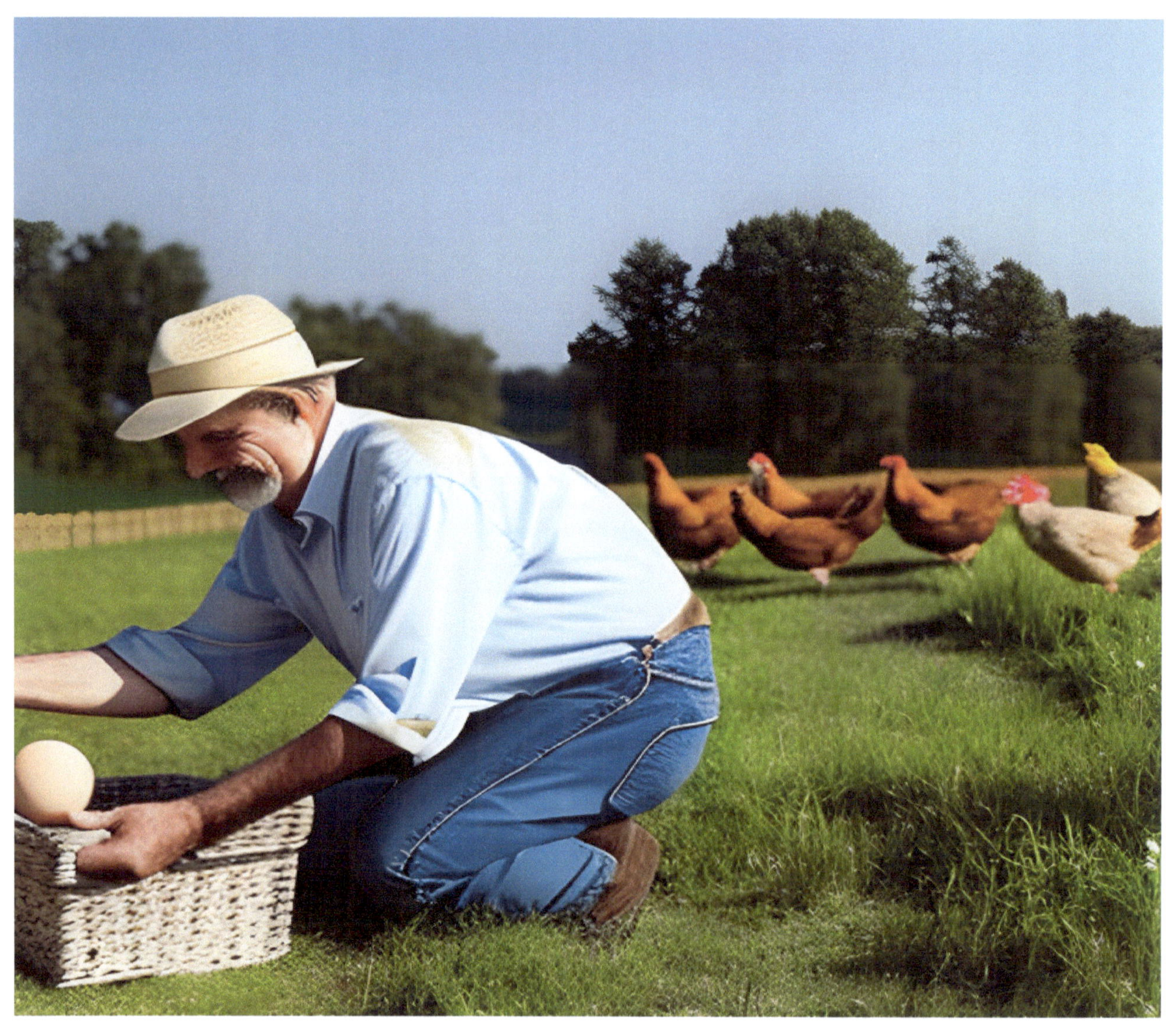

Occasionally the farmer would come around and collect a few eggs.

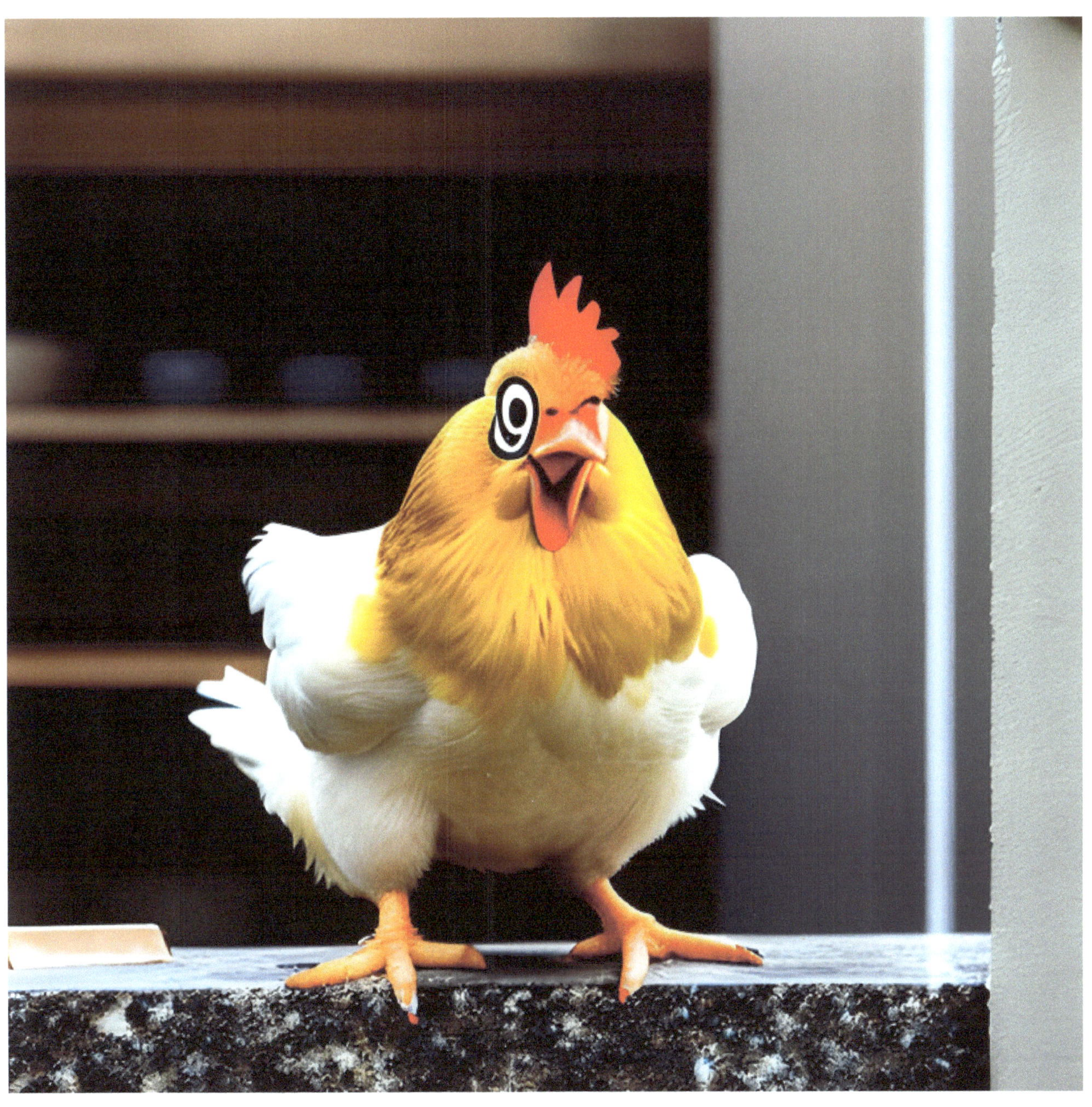

When the farmer tried to take Grace's egg she would squawk and cry. She only had one egg!

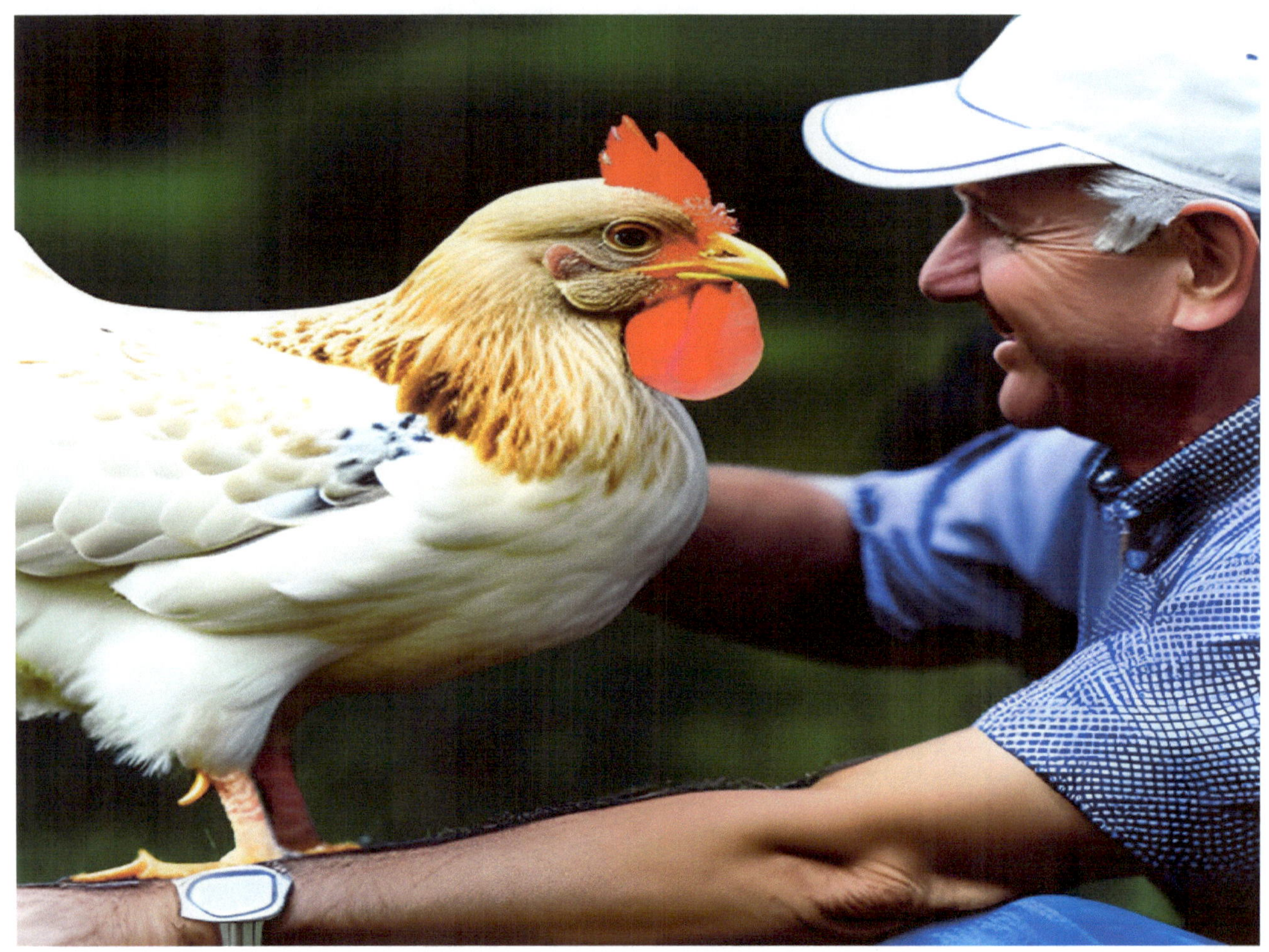

The farmer felt sorry for Grace because he knew how much she wanted to be a mom, so he never took her egg. He would pat her on the head and continue with his duties.

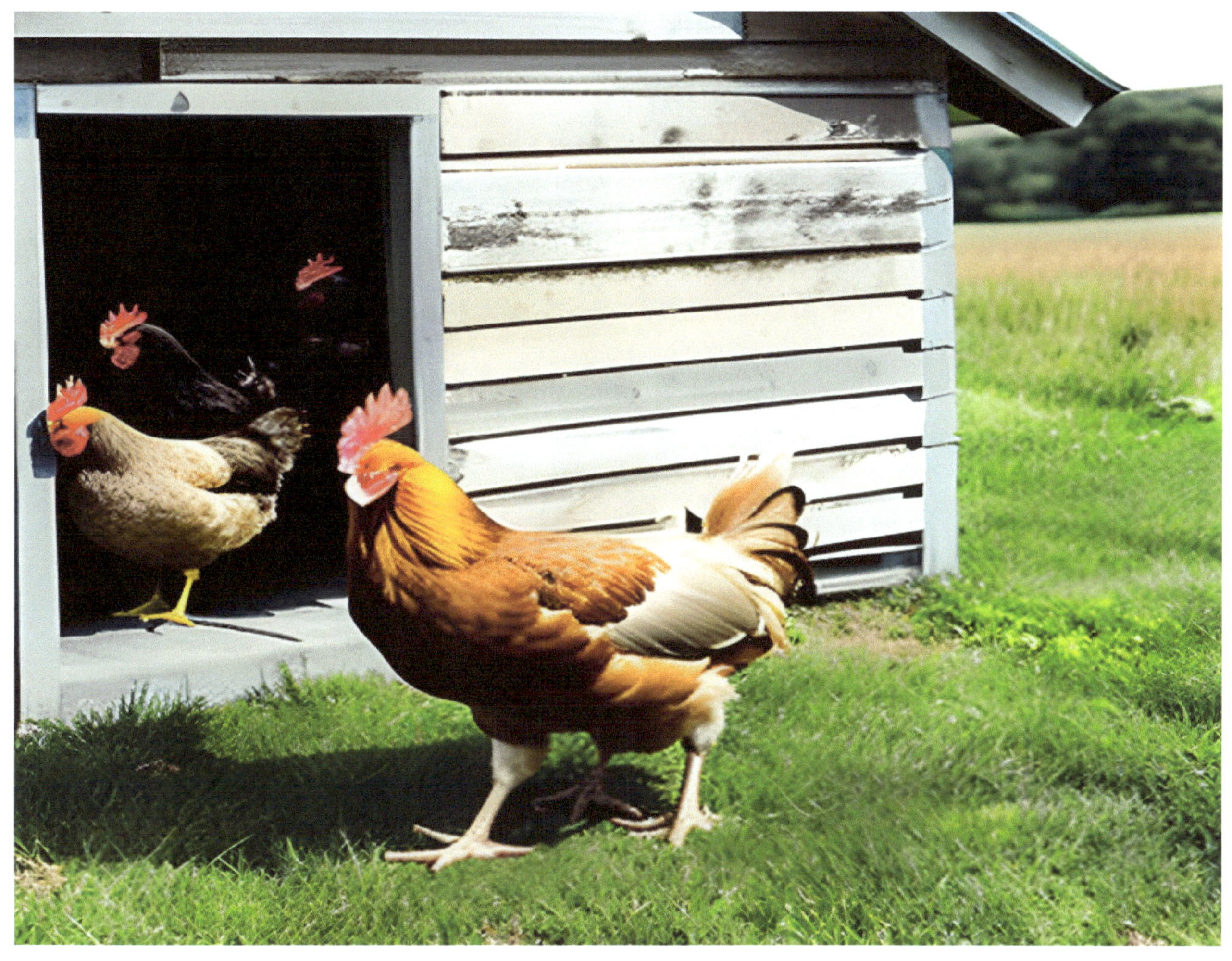

After the farmer collected enough eggs, he would let the chickens out of the hen house so they could eat and play.

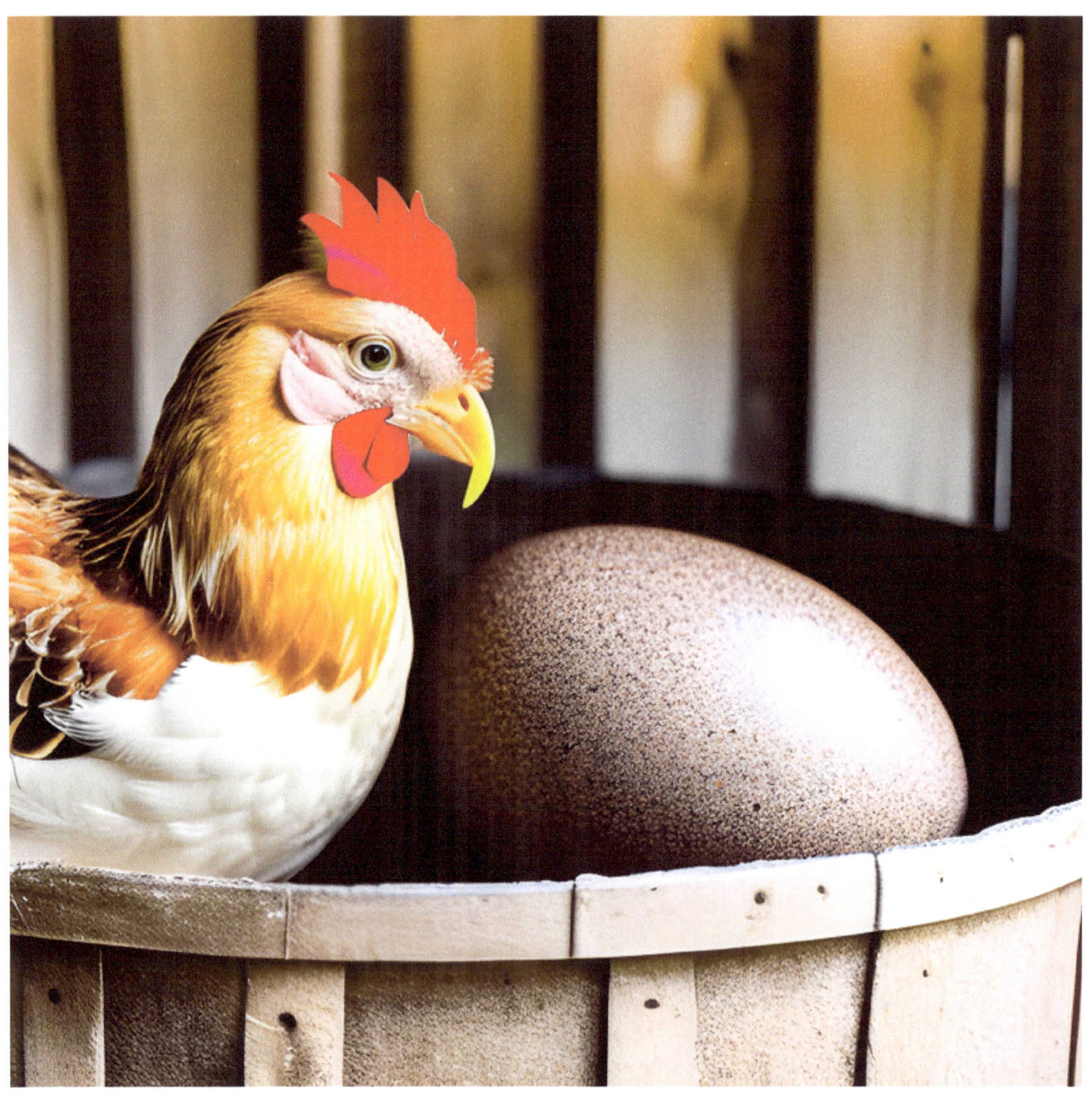

Grace did not go play with the others because she did not want to leave her egg.

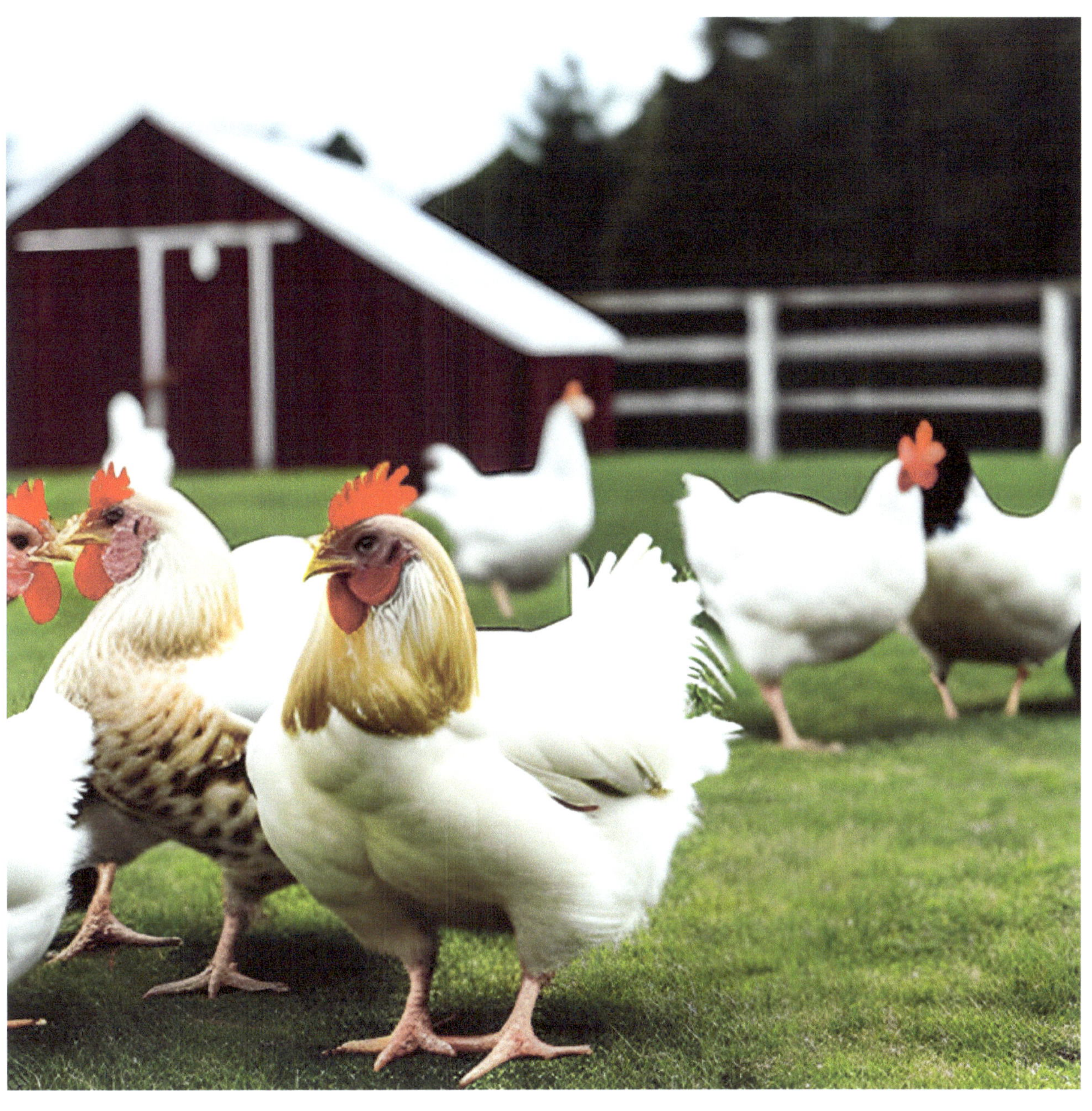

One day Grace needed a break from sitting on her egg. She did not see the farmer, so she got up to stretch her legs and visit with her friends and play with their chicks.

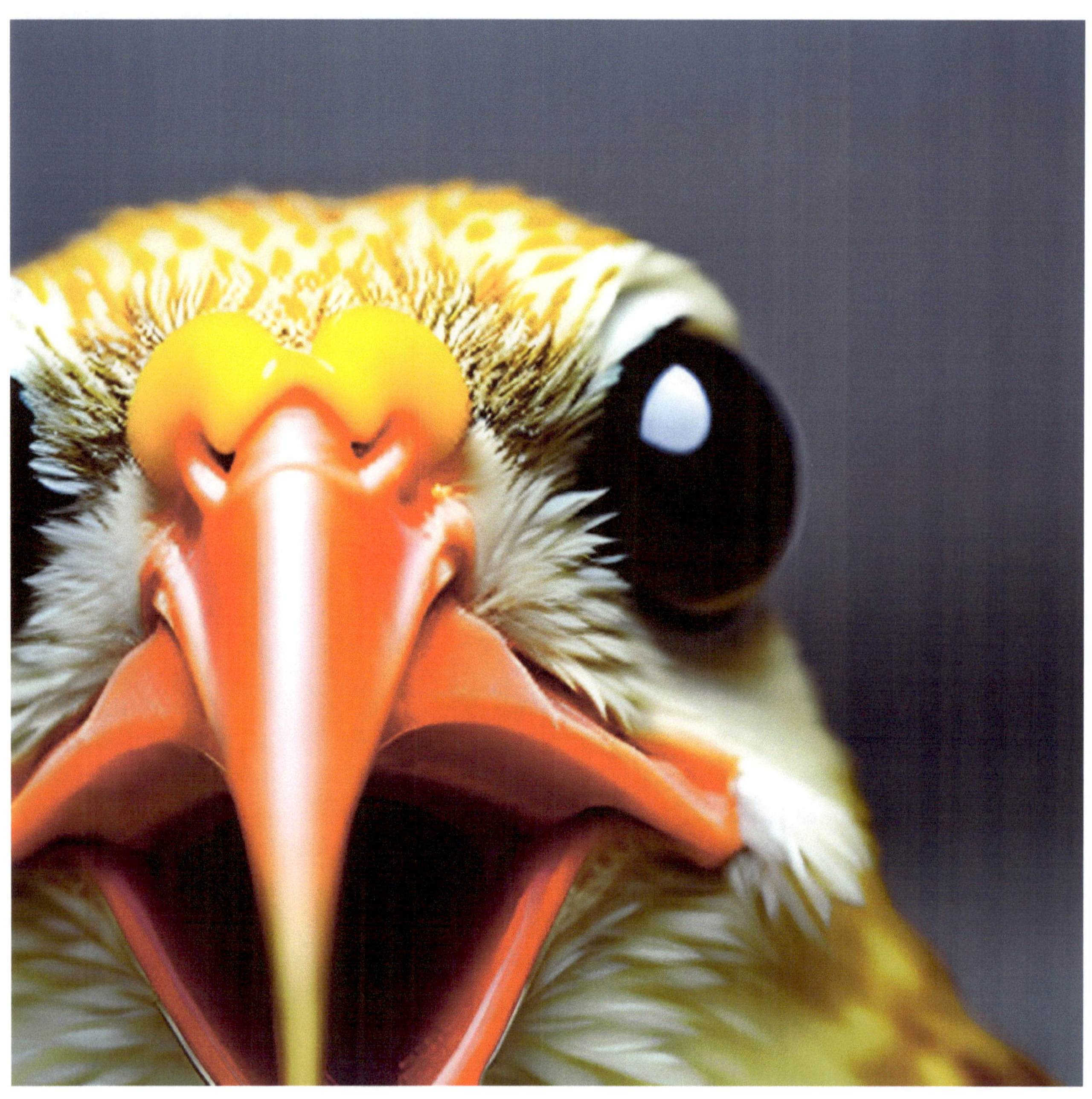

Grace was having such a good time with her friends she forgot about her egg!

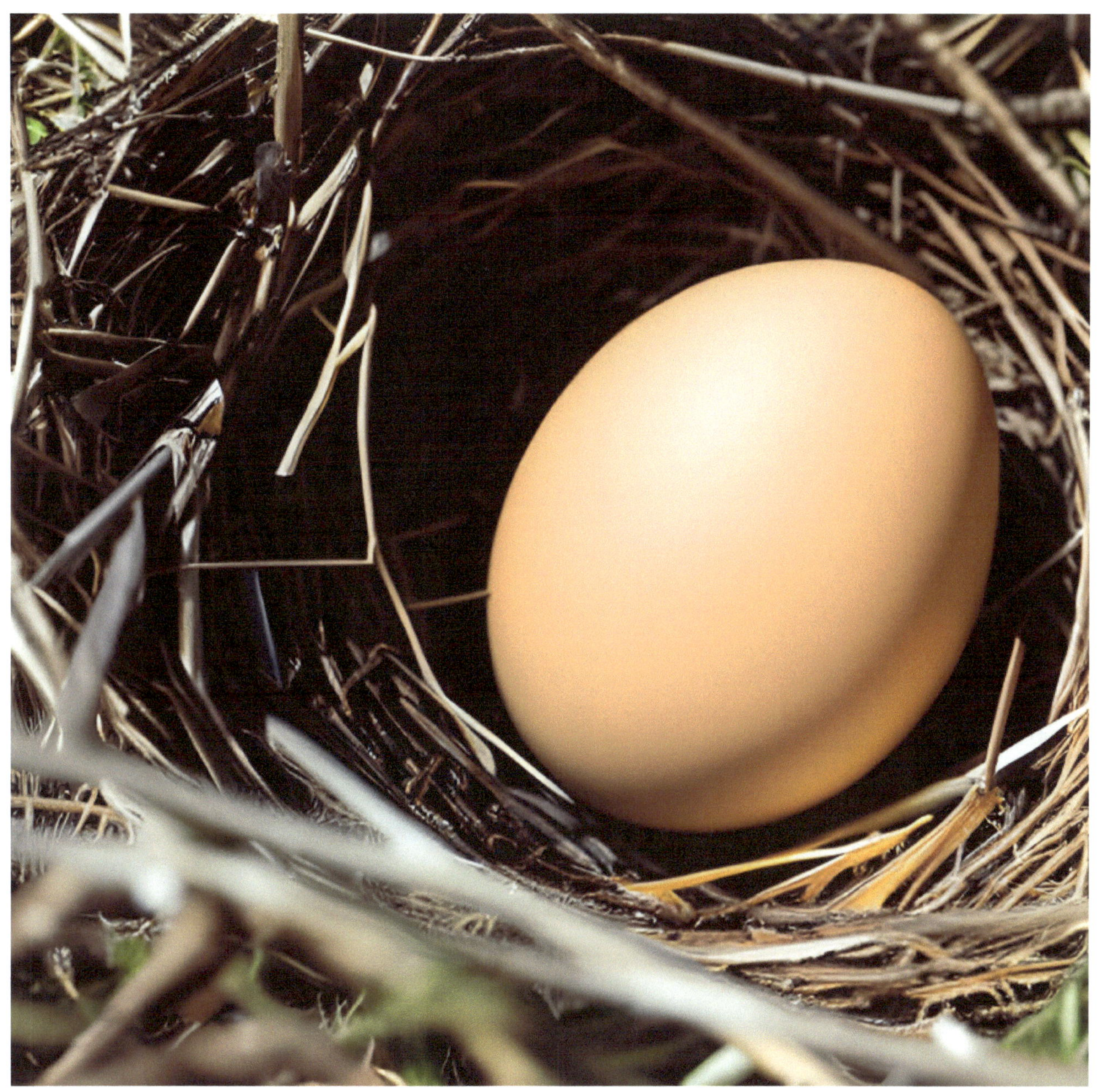

Grace remembered her egg and hurried back to the hen house. When she arrived, her egg was still there, but she decided to hide her egg the next time she decided to leave.

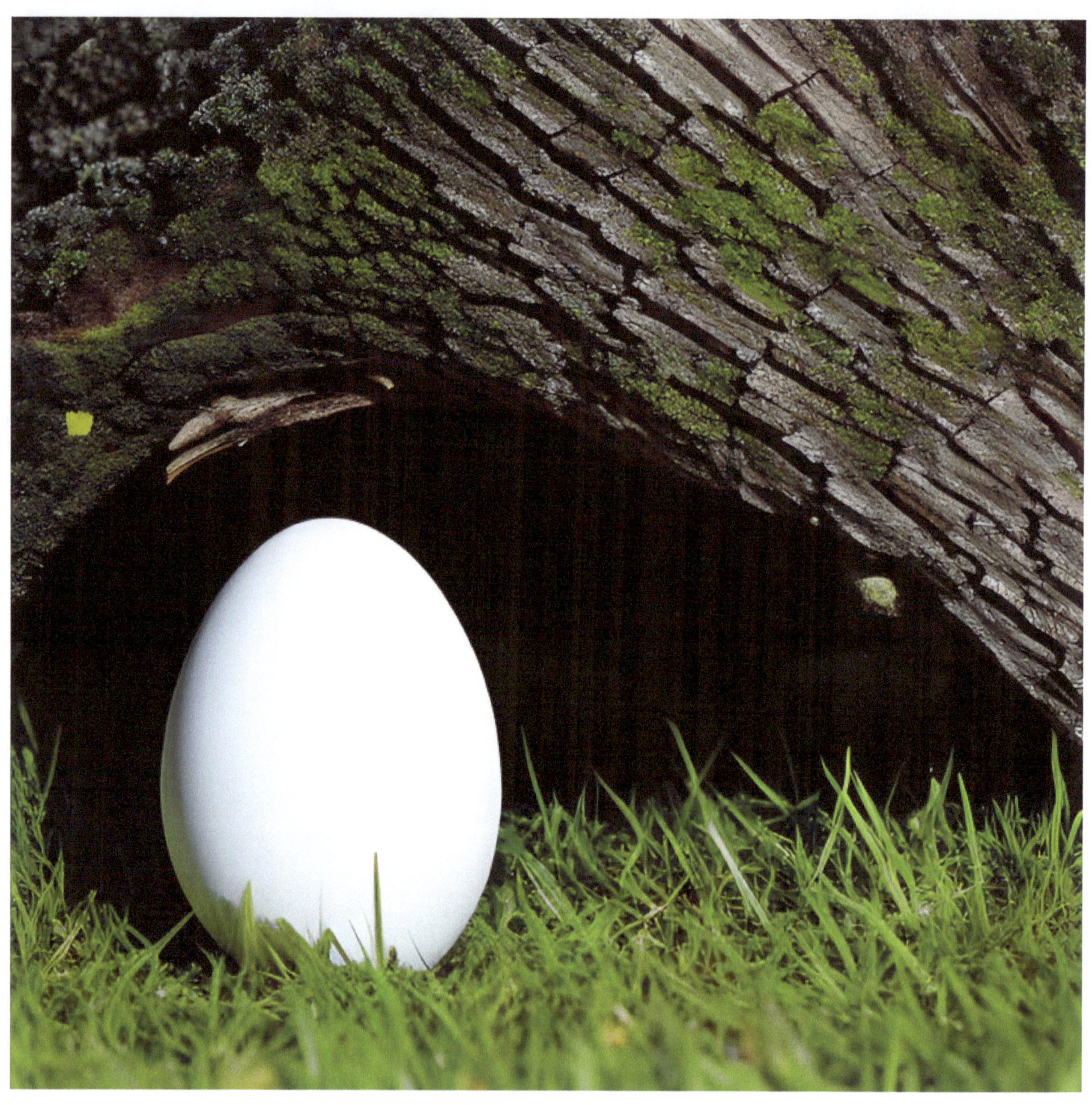

The next time Grace went to play with the other hens and their chicks in the barnyard she hid her egg.

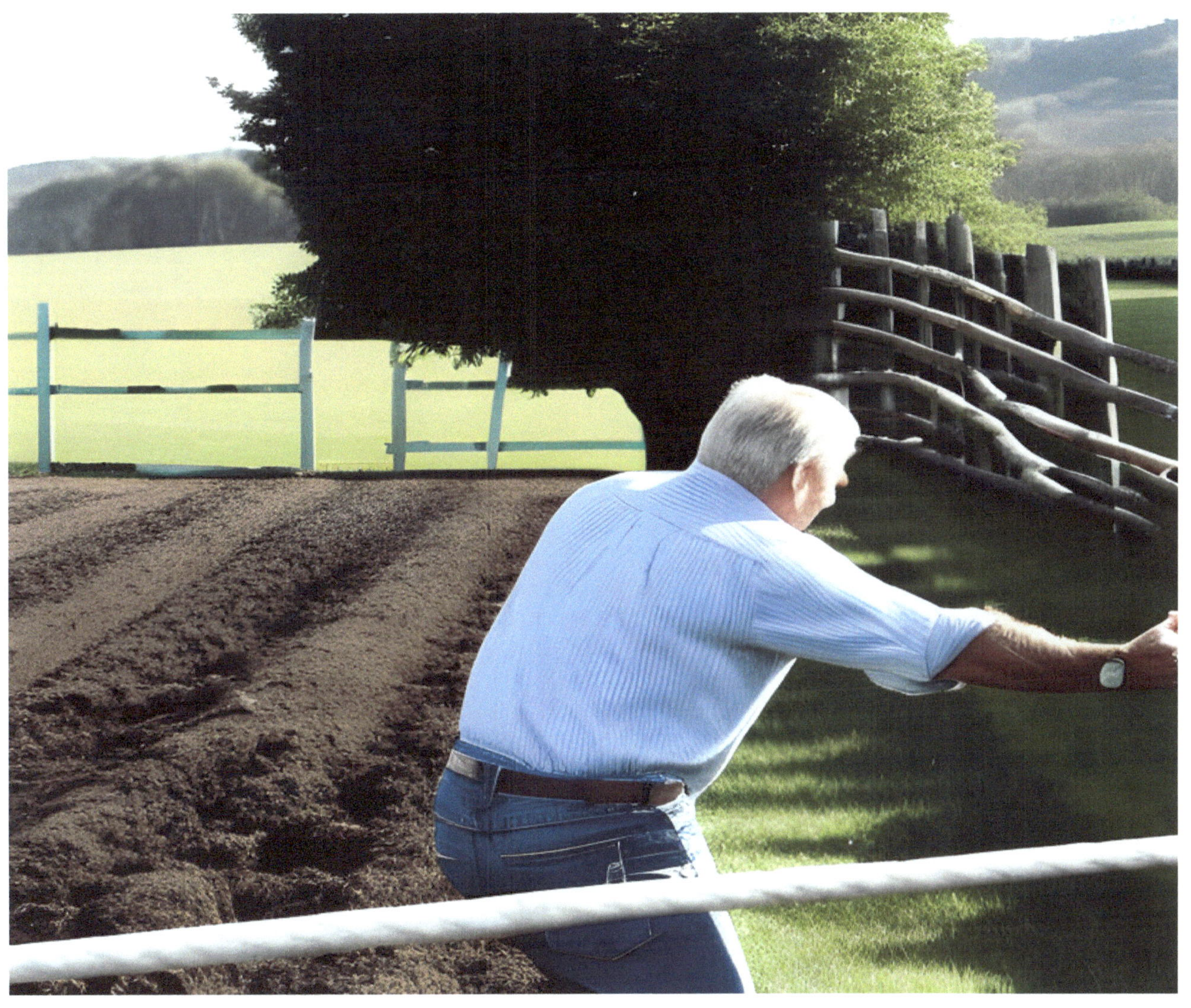

The farmer watched as Grace hid her beloved
egg. He knew the egg was not going to hatch and
was going to rot. He didn't want Grace to see the
rotten egg, so he threw it over the fence.

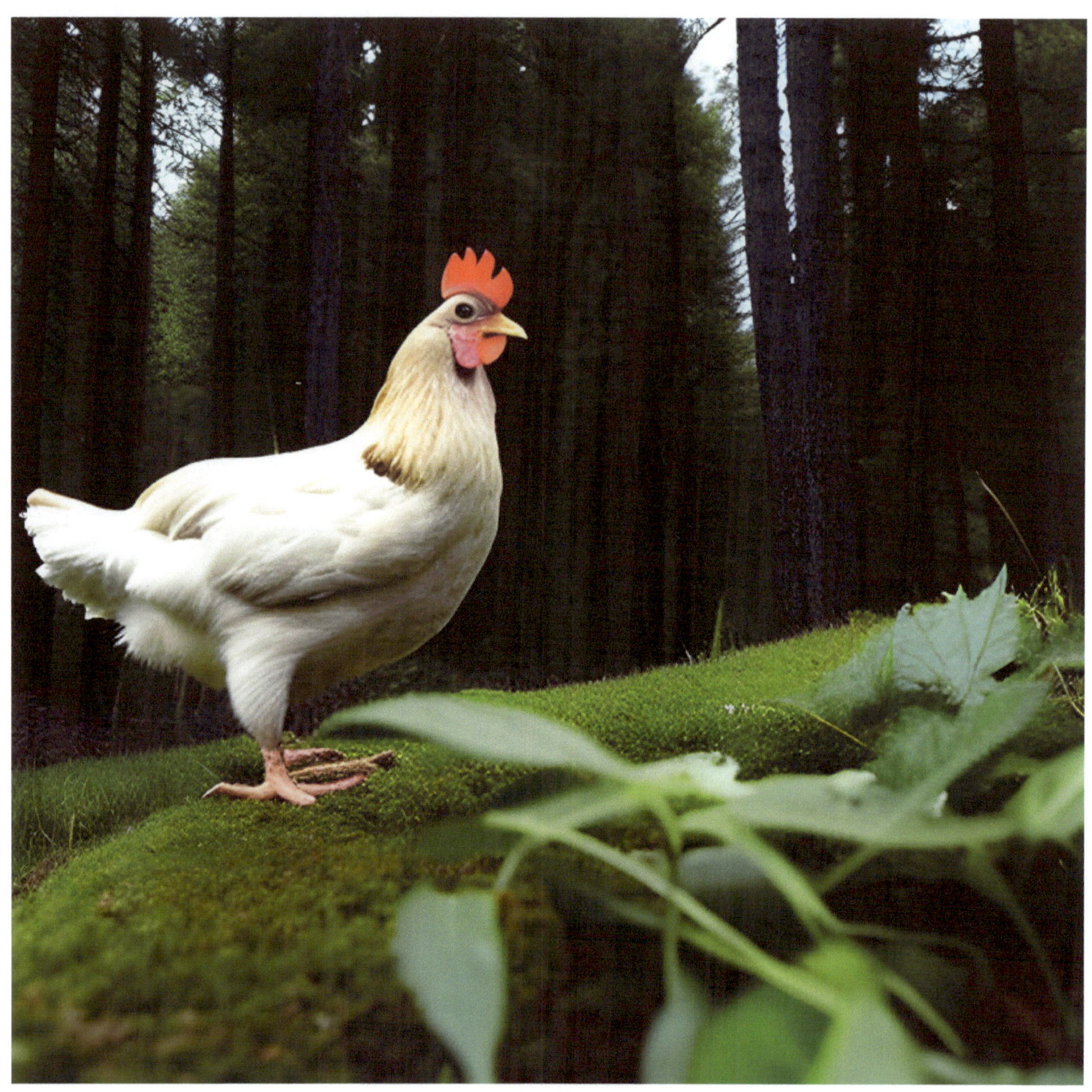

When Grace was finished in the barnyard she
went back to search for her egg. She looked and
looked but could not find it.

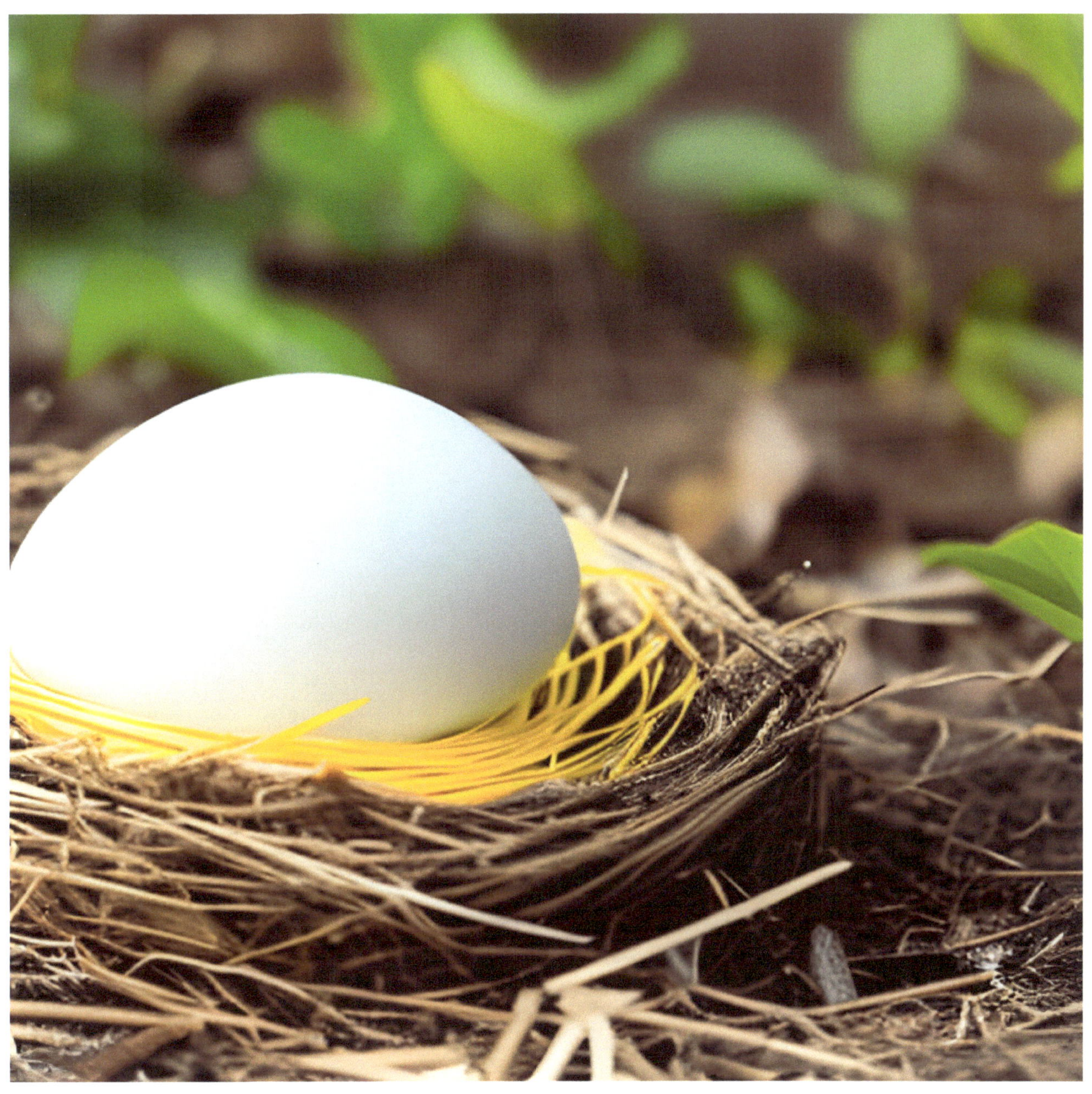

Grace went back to the hen house crying because she couldn't find her egg. To her surprise the next day she laid a new egg!!!!

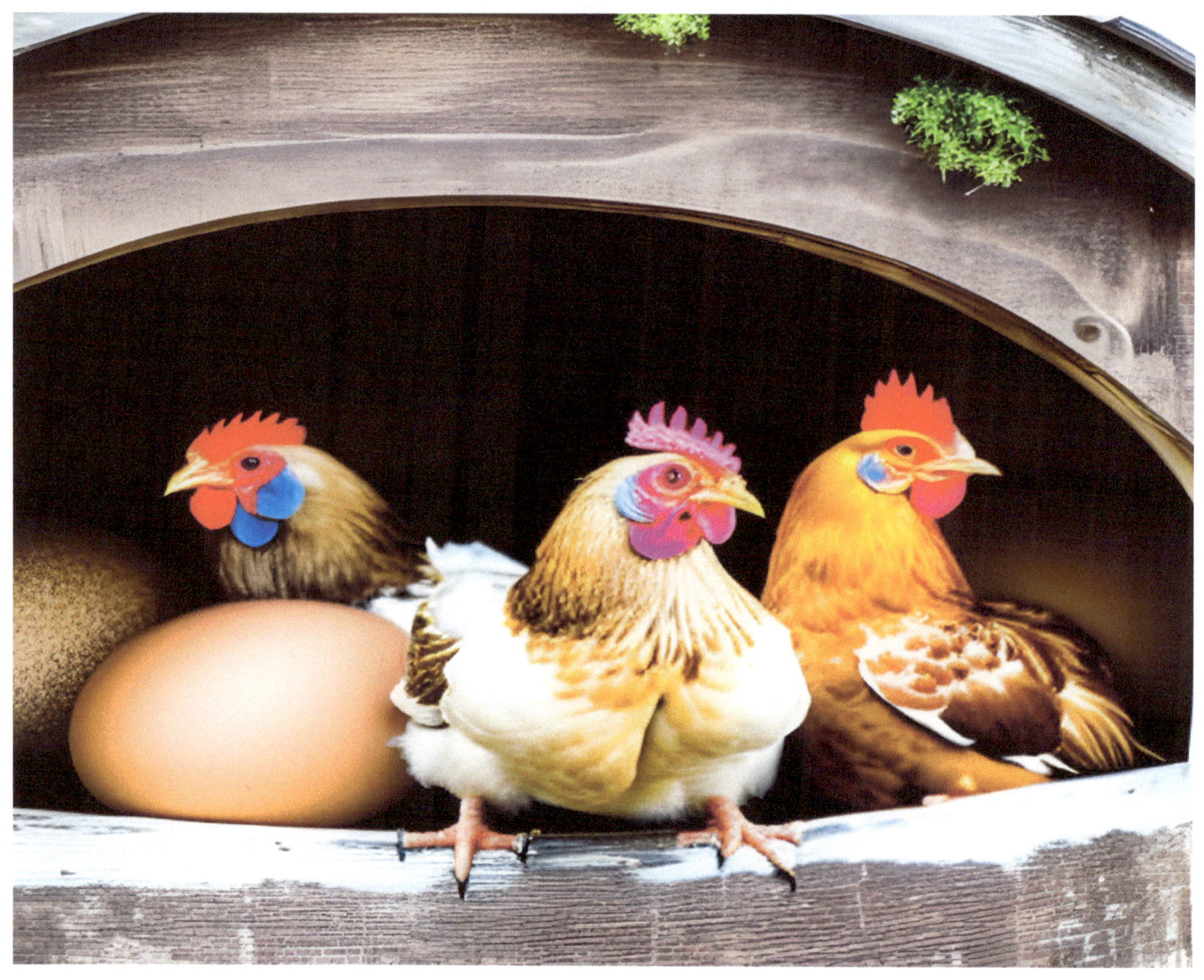

Grace was especially happy because her friend laid an egg the same day she did! She could already picture their chicks playing together in the barnyard.

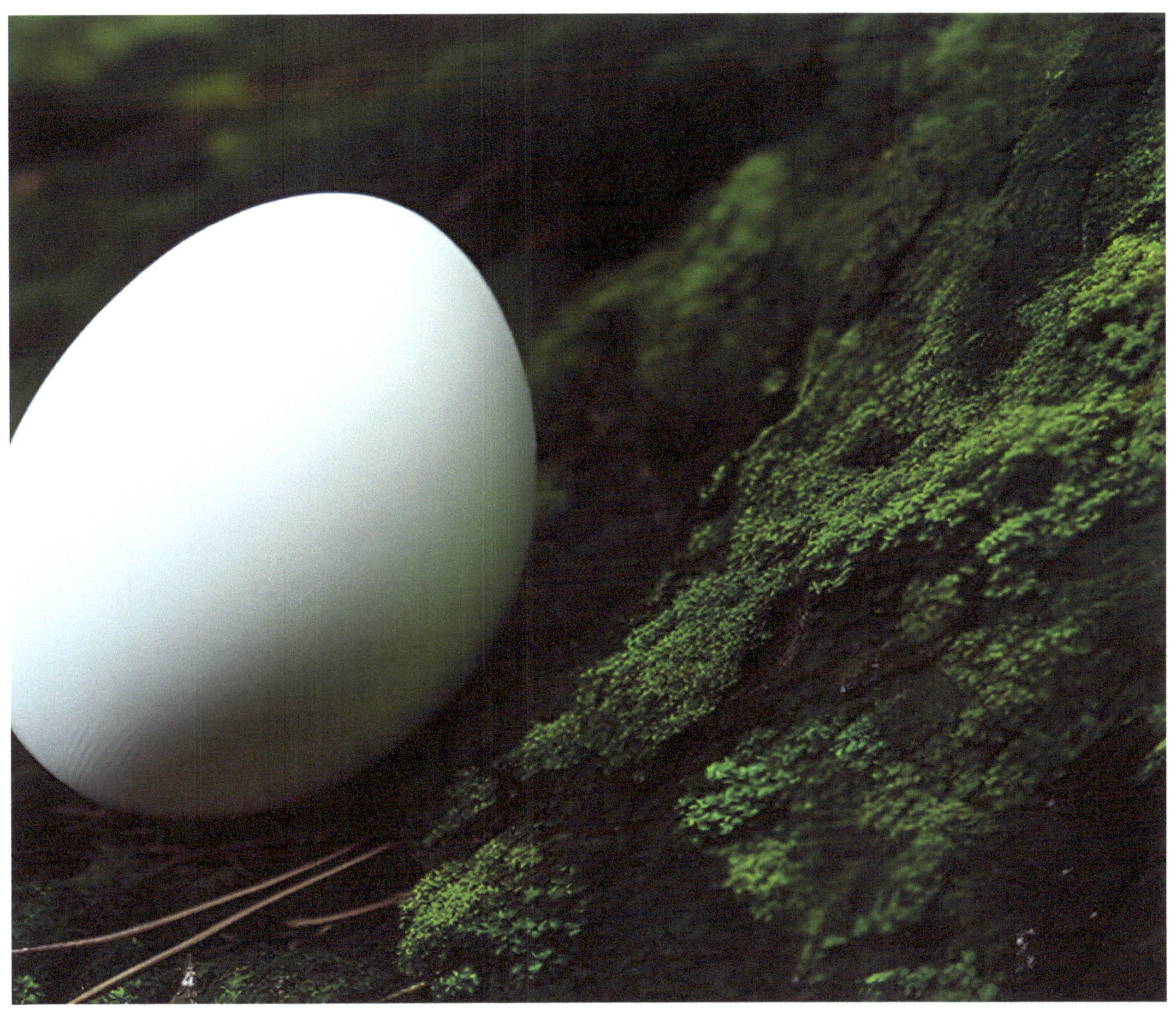

The days went by, and her friend's egg hatched, but Grace was still waiting for her egg to hatch. She had been sitting on her egg so long she needed a break. She decided to hide her beloved egg under a tree while she visited the barnyard.

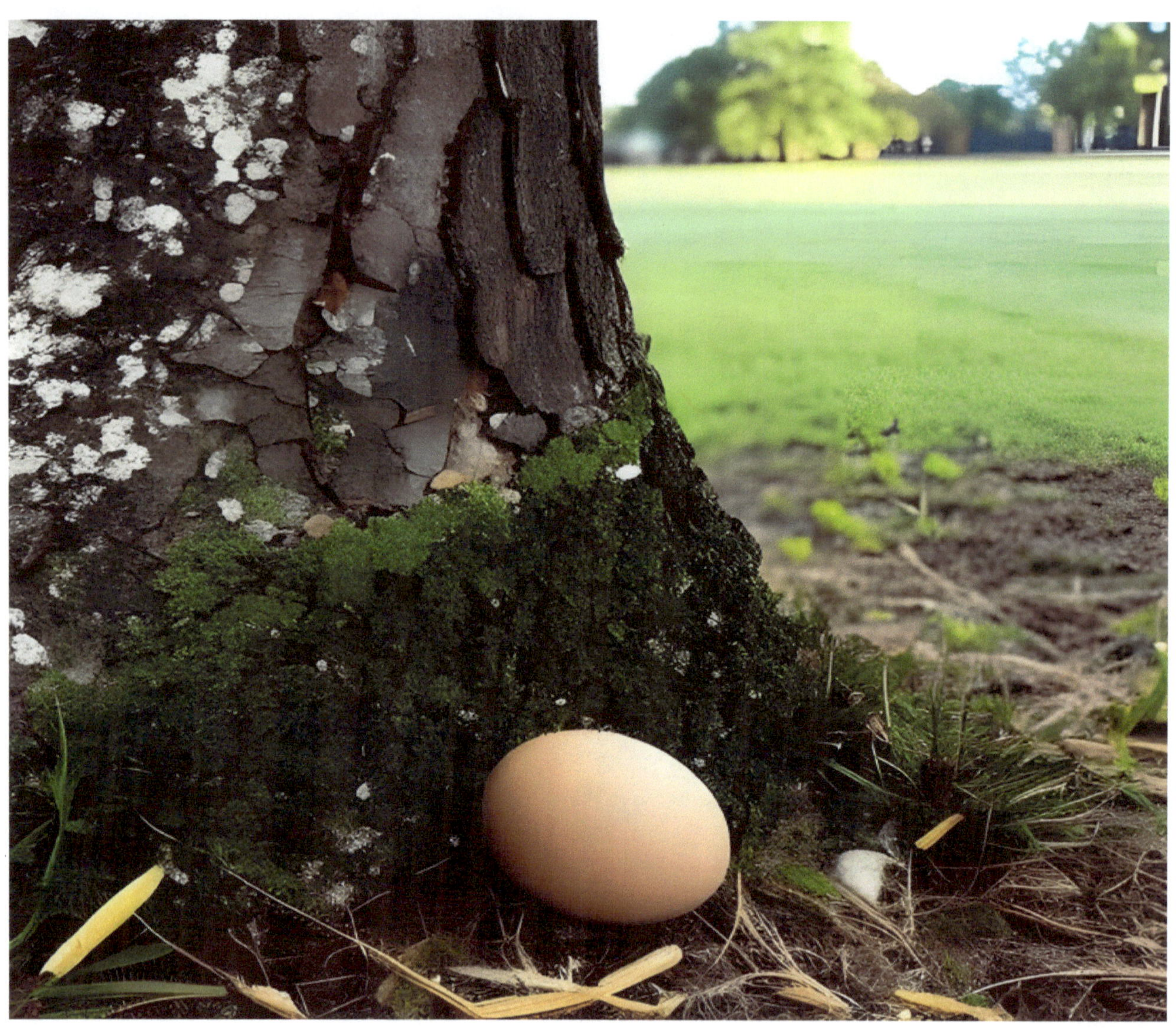

The farmer once again saw Grace hiding her egg. He went to check on the egg and saw it was rotting. He didn't want Grace to see her egg was rotting and threw this egg over the fence too.

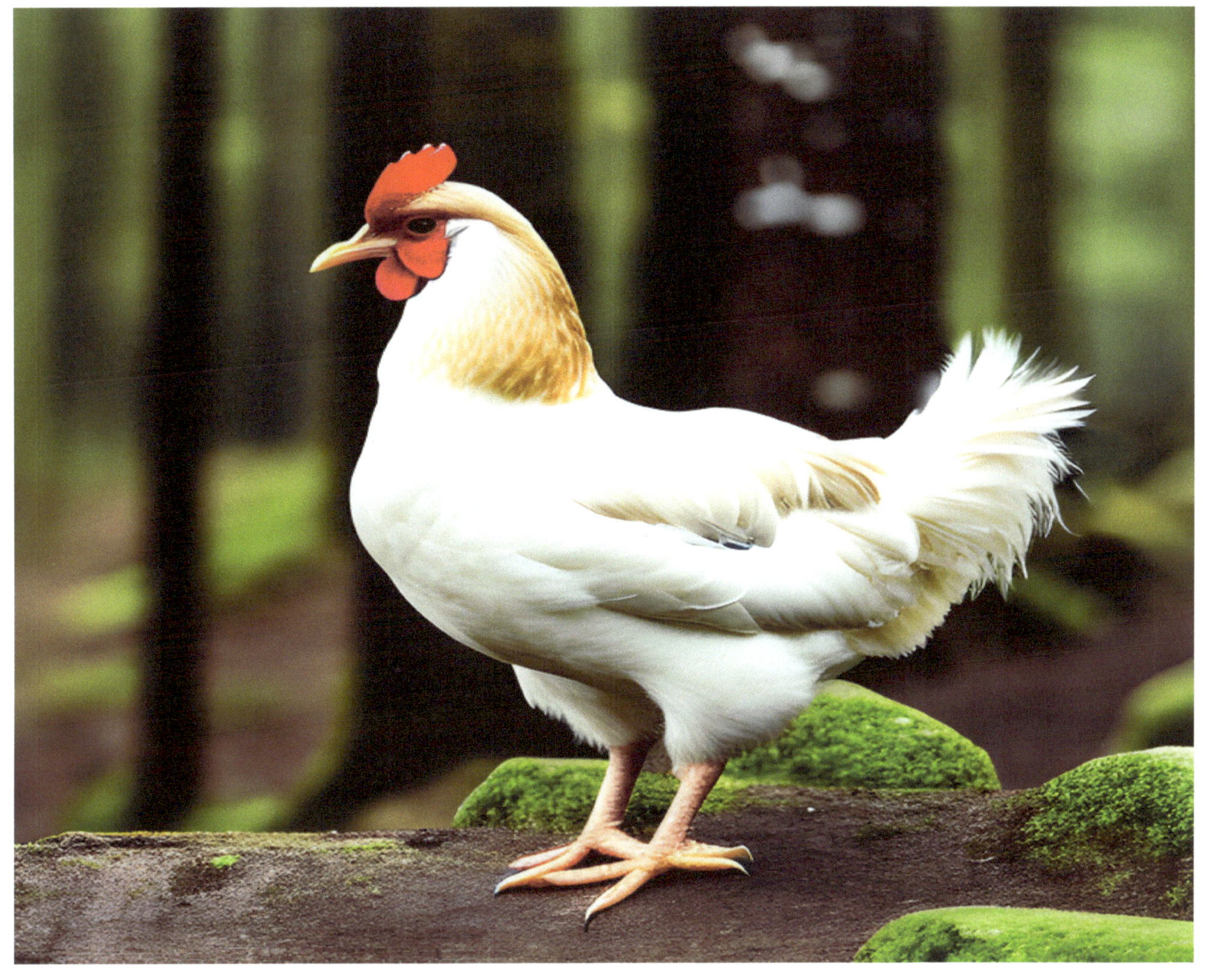

Grace came back from the barnyard and looked everywhere for her egg. To her dismay she could not find it.

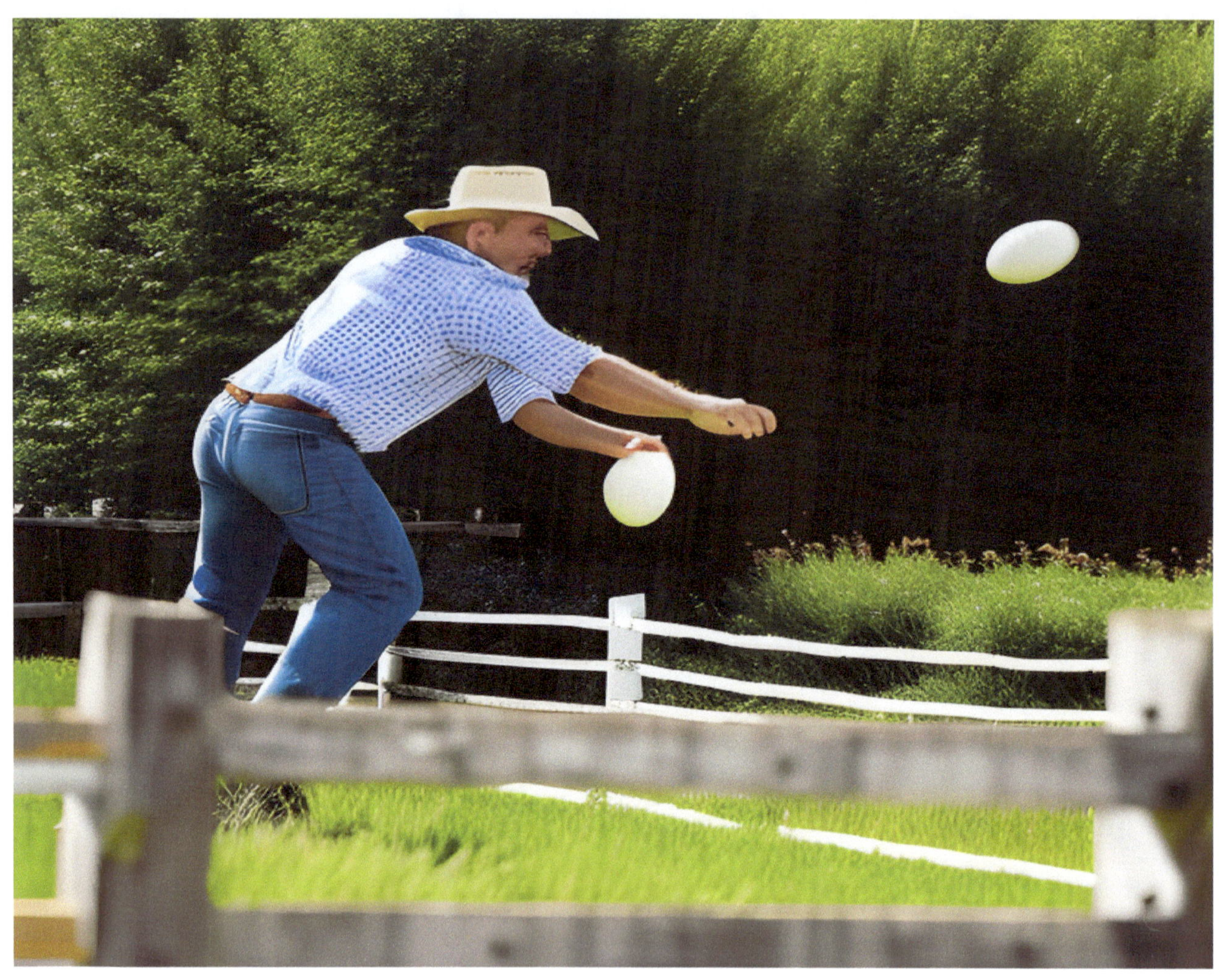

As the years went by Grace continued to hide her egg whenever she needed a break. The farmer continued to watch her and threw the rotten eggs over the fence.

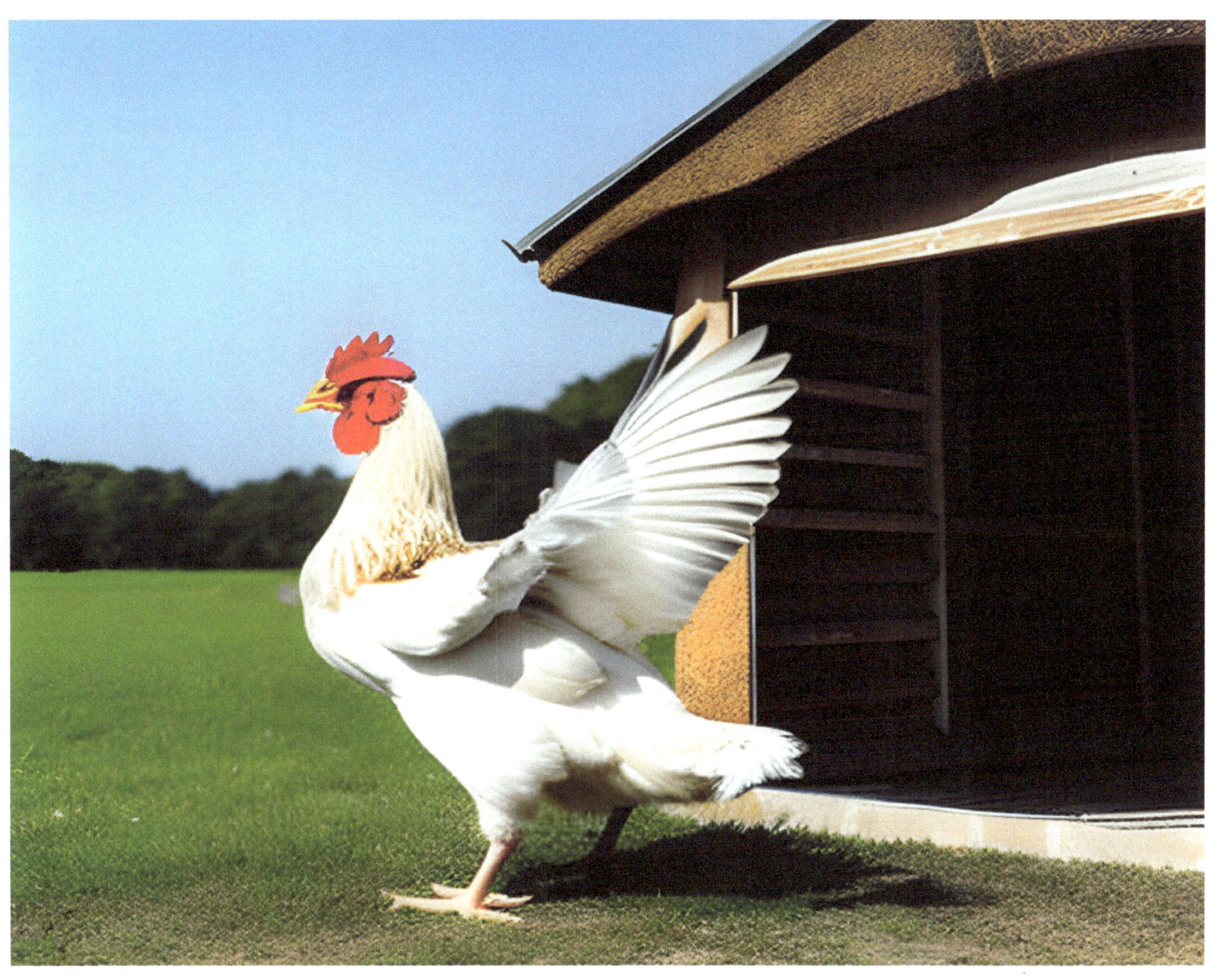

Grace never gave up her dream of being a mom and continued to hide her eggs and cry if the farmer tried to take her rotting egg.

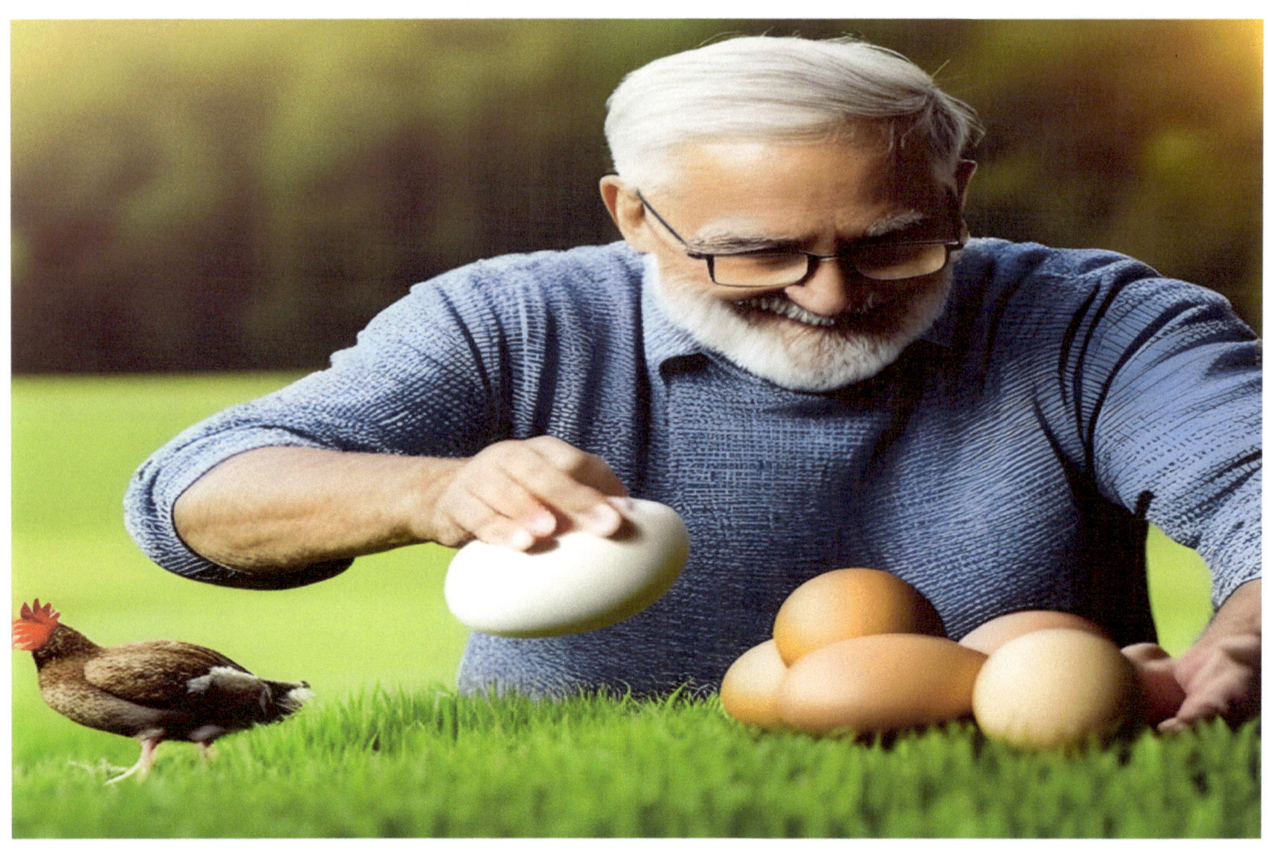

One day the farmer finished collecting eggs from the ducks and headed into the hen house. He saw Grace sitting on her egg and suddenly decided to switch her egg with one of the duck eggs he had just collected in his bucket. Grace cried as he lifted her up and then she happily sat back down on her egg. She had no idea her egg had been replaced with a duck egg!

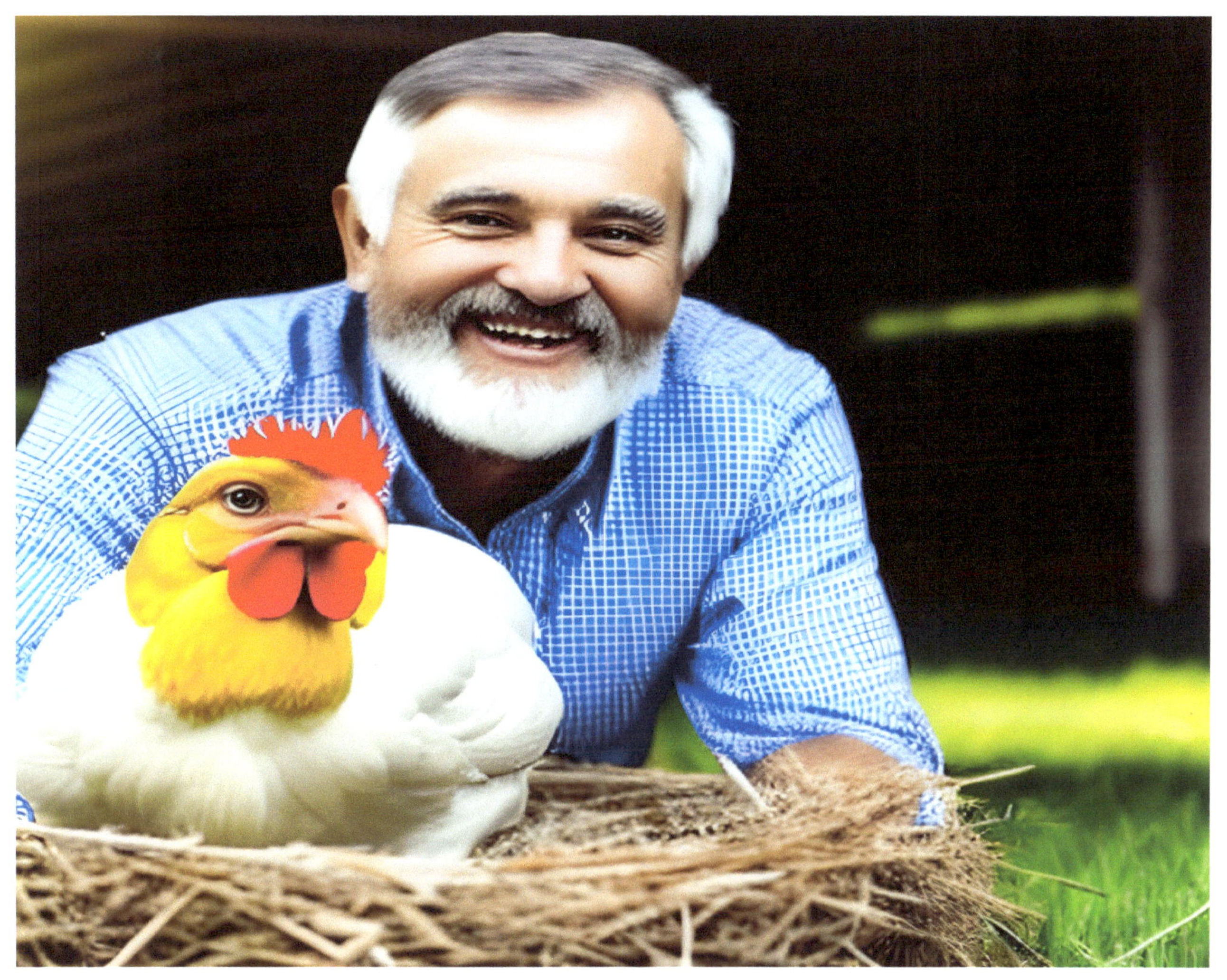

The days went by, and Grace stayed on her beloved egg and never left it. The farmer checked on her every day and was happy to see that she may have a chick of her own soon.

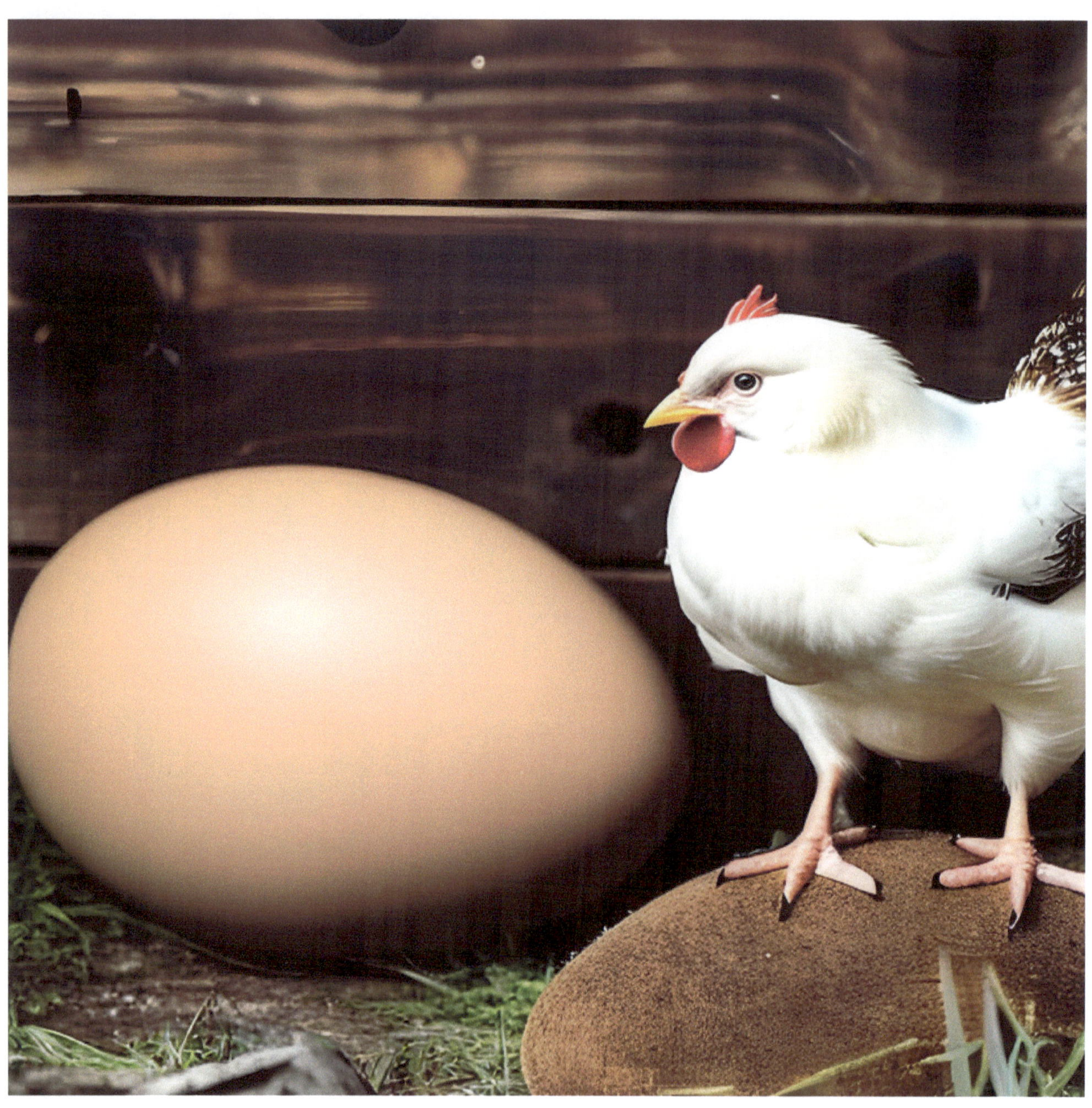

The days got closer and any day now Grace was FINALLY going to see her dream come true!

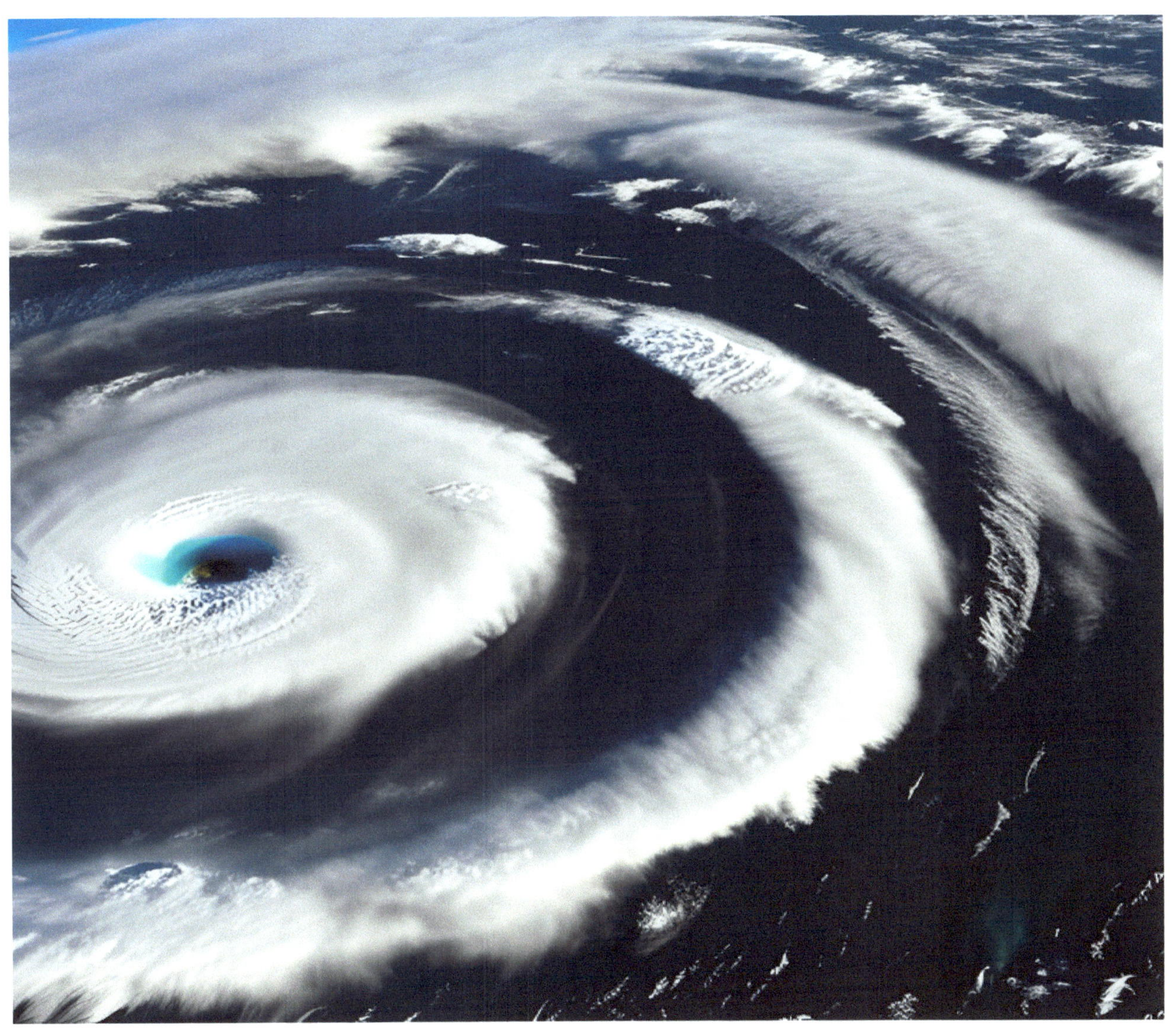

In 2004, a category 4 hurricane hit Florida called Hurricane Frances. Everyone was told to evacuate from this devastating storm.

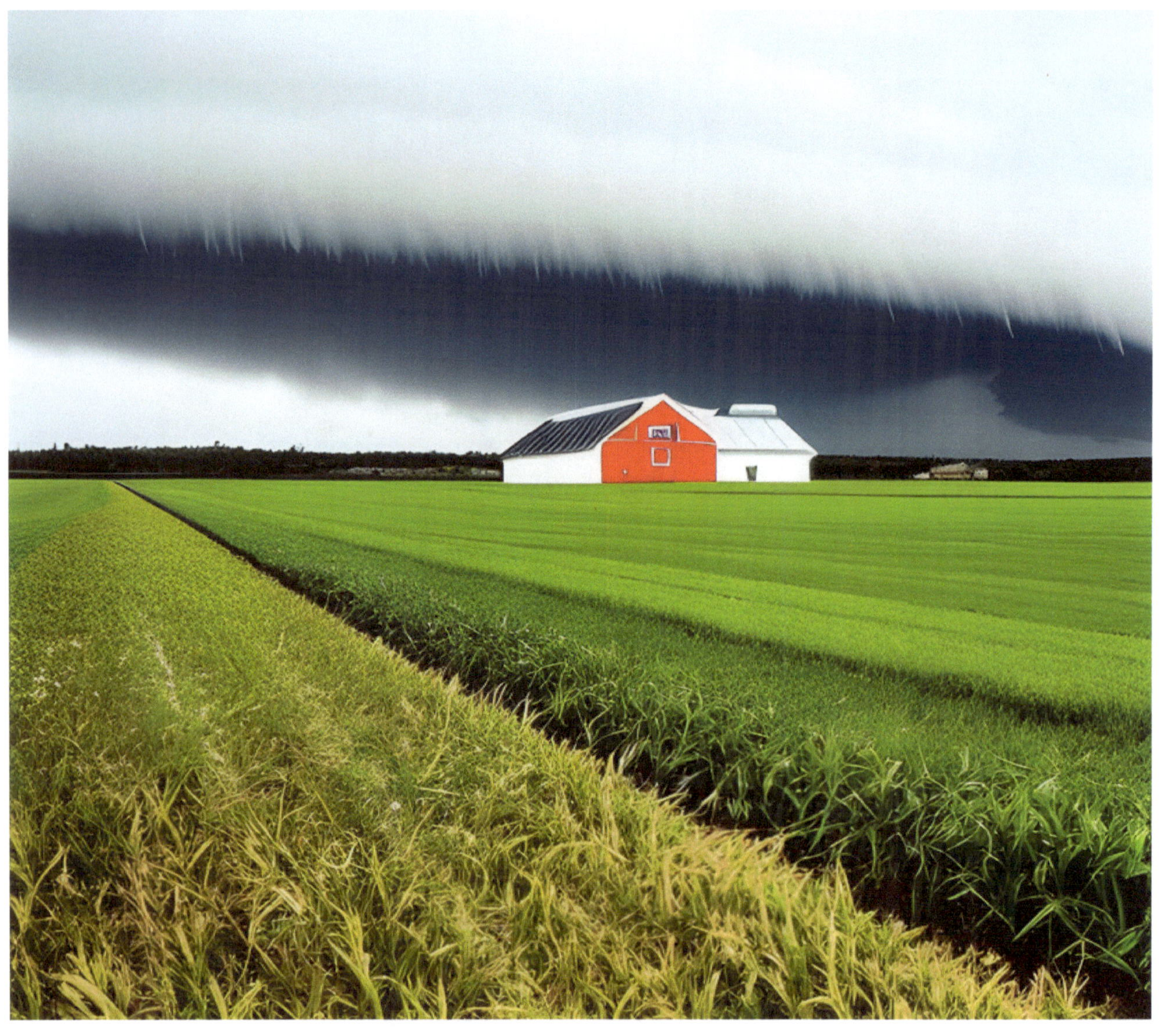

The farmer secured his farm for the storm and took one last look around his farm to ensure the livestock was locked in and safe. On his way to his truck, he happened to glance at the hen house and thought of Grace. He decided at the last minute to check on her as the winds tore through the air.

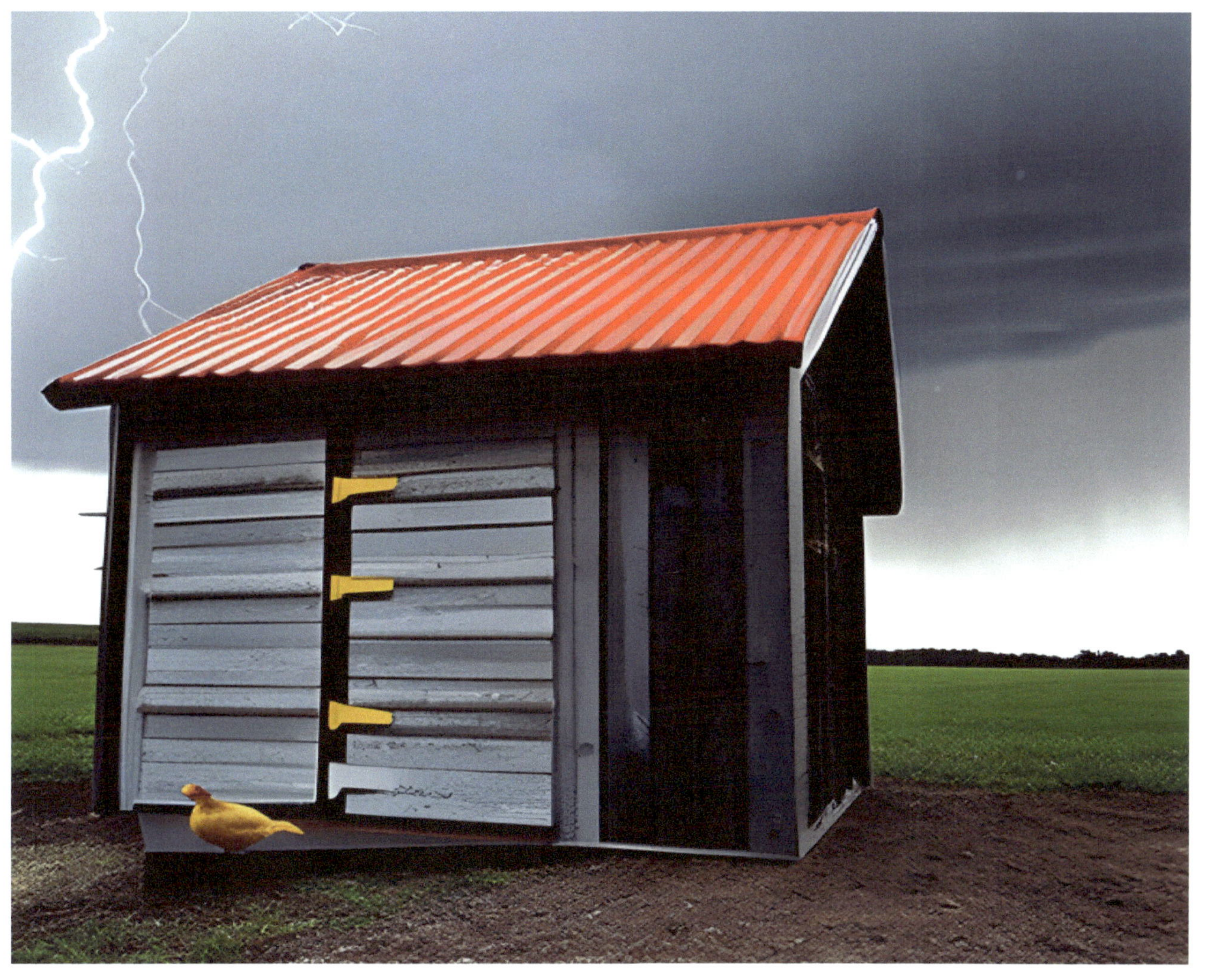

As he looked in the hen house, he saw Grace hunkering down with her egg. He locked up the hen house and drove away from the farm as the hurricane force winds whipped through it.

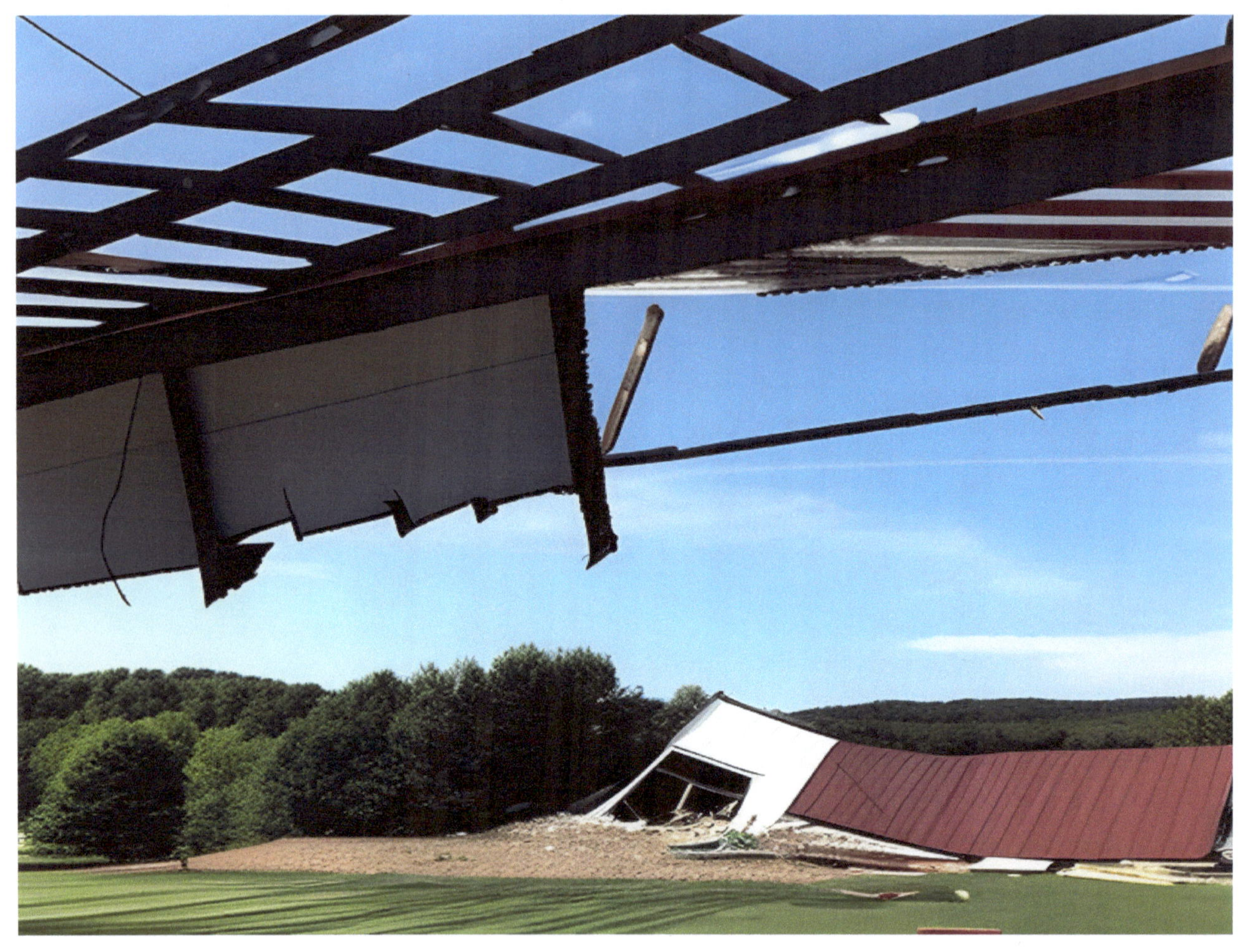

The farmer came back to his farm the next day and saw devastation. The first thing he did was check on the animals.

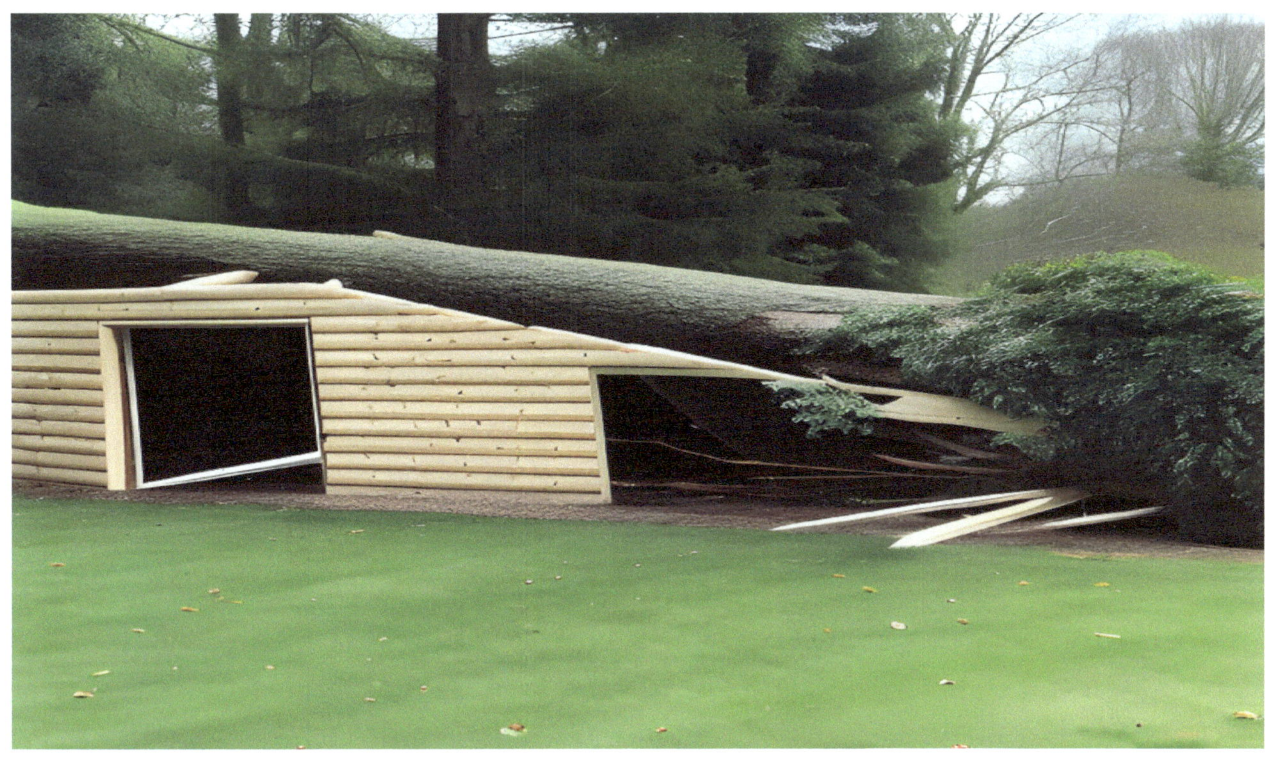

A tree had fallen on the hen house and the farmer had tears in his eyes. He raced to the hen house and found all the hens were okay, but he could not find Grace. The tree had hit the spot she usually stayed in. He looked all over the hen house and finally found her hiding under some wood and debris.

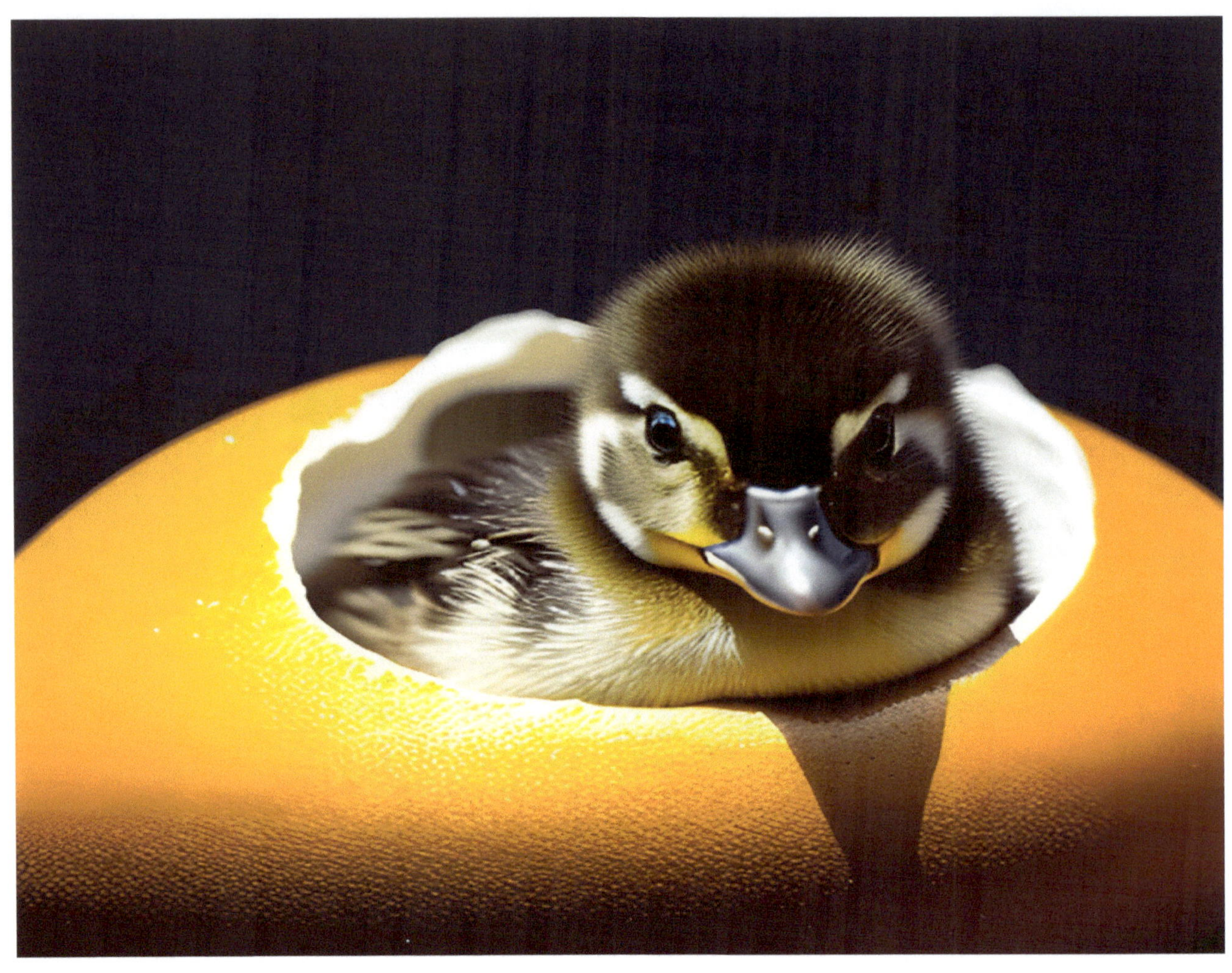

Grace must have moved her egg one last time...

The farmer pulled the debris away and to his shock he saw Grace with a newly born hatchling. He knew right away its name was going to be Frances since she was born during Hurricane Frances.

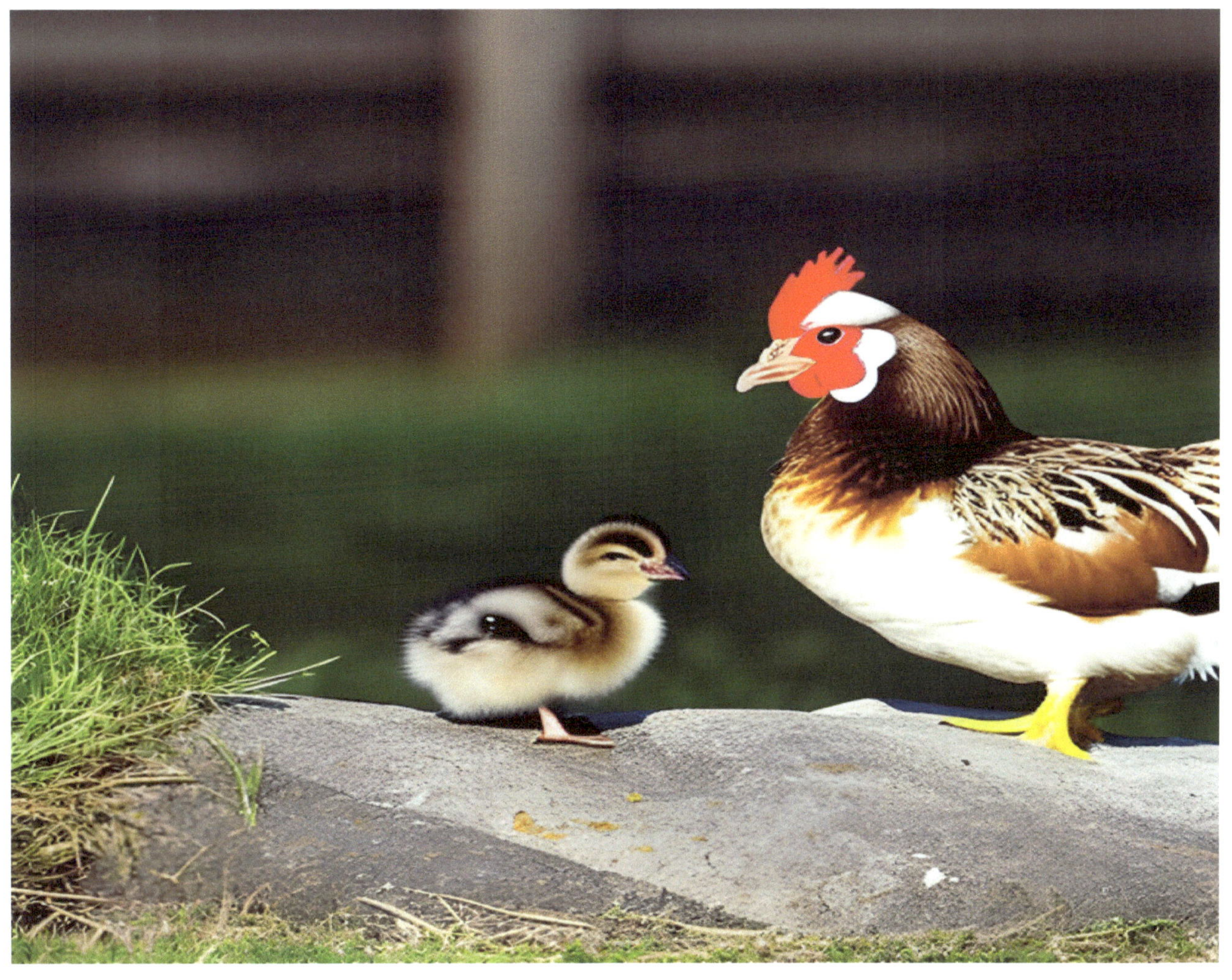

The farmer fixed up the farm over the next several days. While he was fixing his farm he smiled as he saw Grace and Frances together in the barnyard.

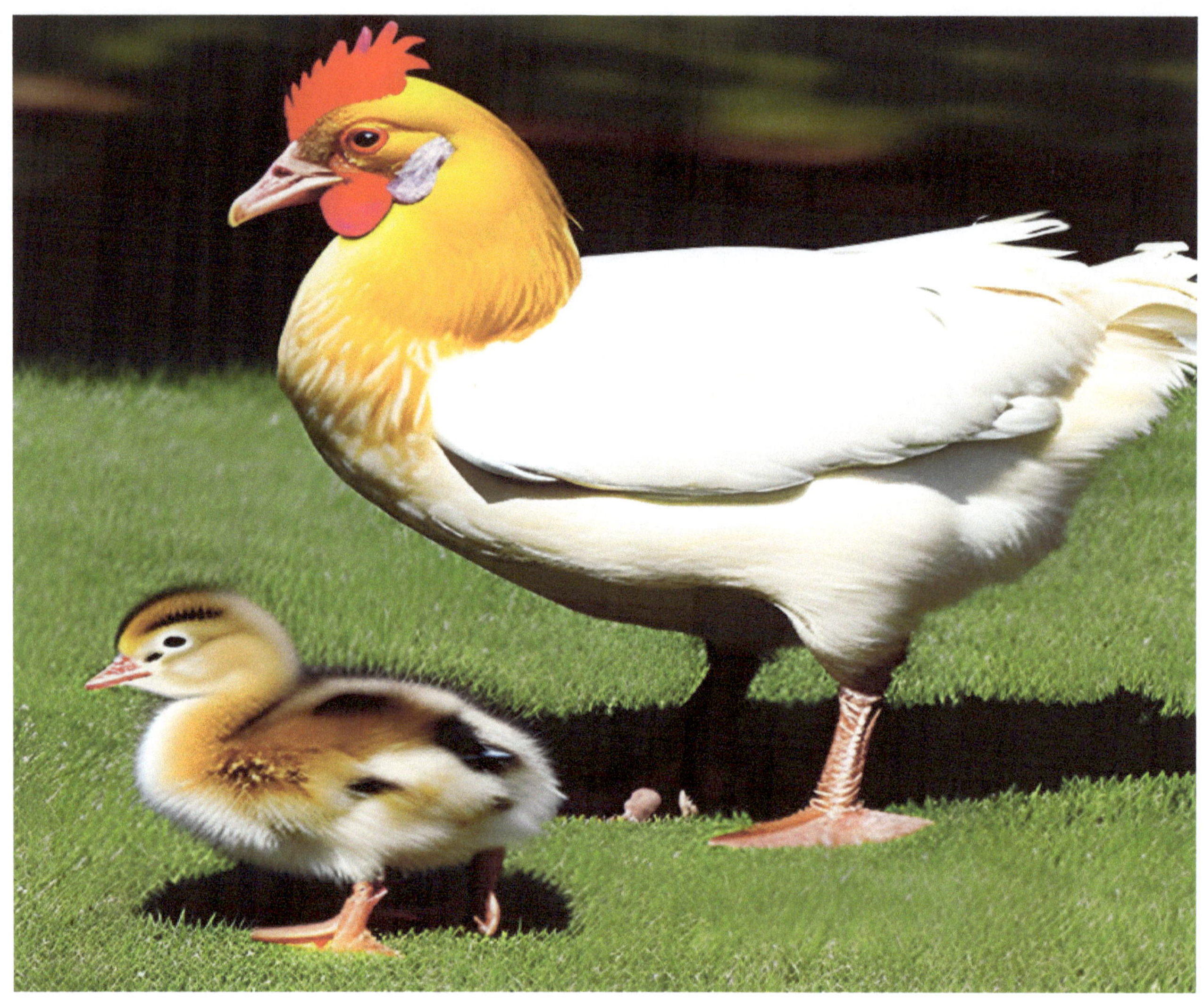

Grace was finally a mom. She loved Frances, the baby duckling, as her own from the moment Frances was hatched. The farmer was overjoyed to see Frances following Grace all over the farm.

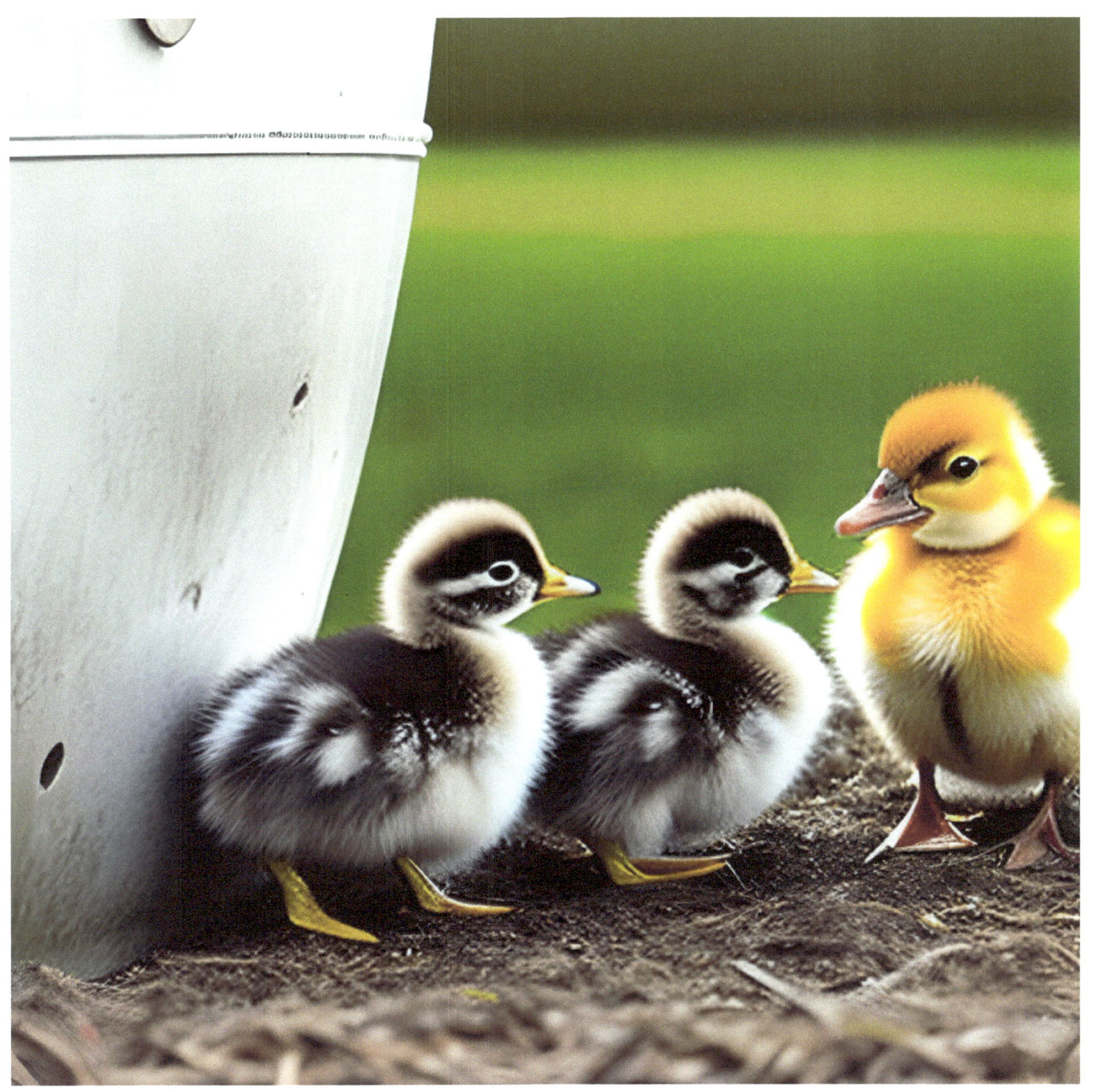

Frances would fall right in line with all the other chicks.

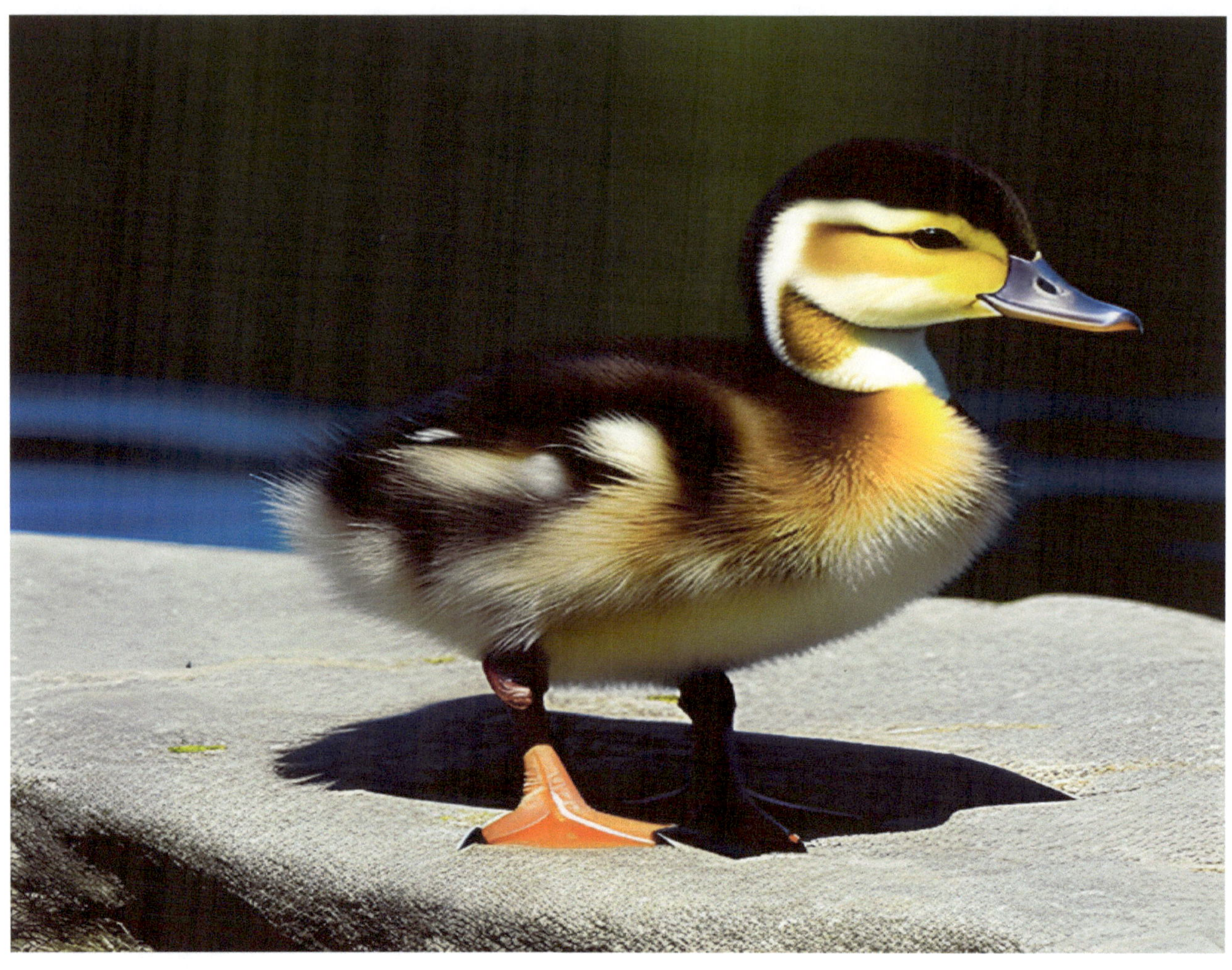

Frances grew into a beautiful duck, but still stayed with Grace and the other hens. Frances could have easily gone over to the ducks, but never did. She knew who her mother was.

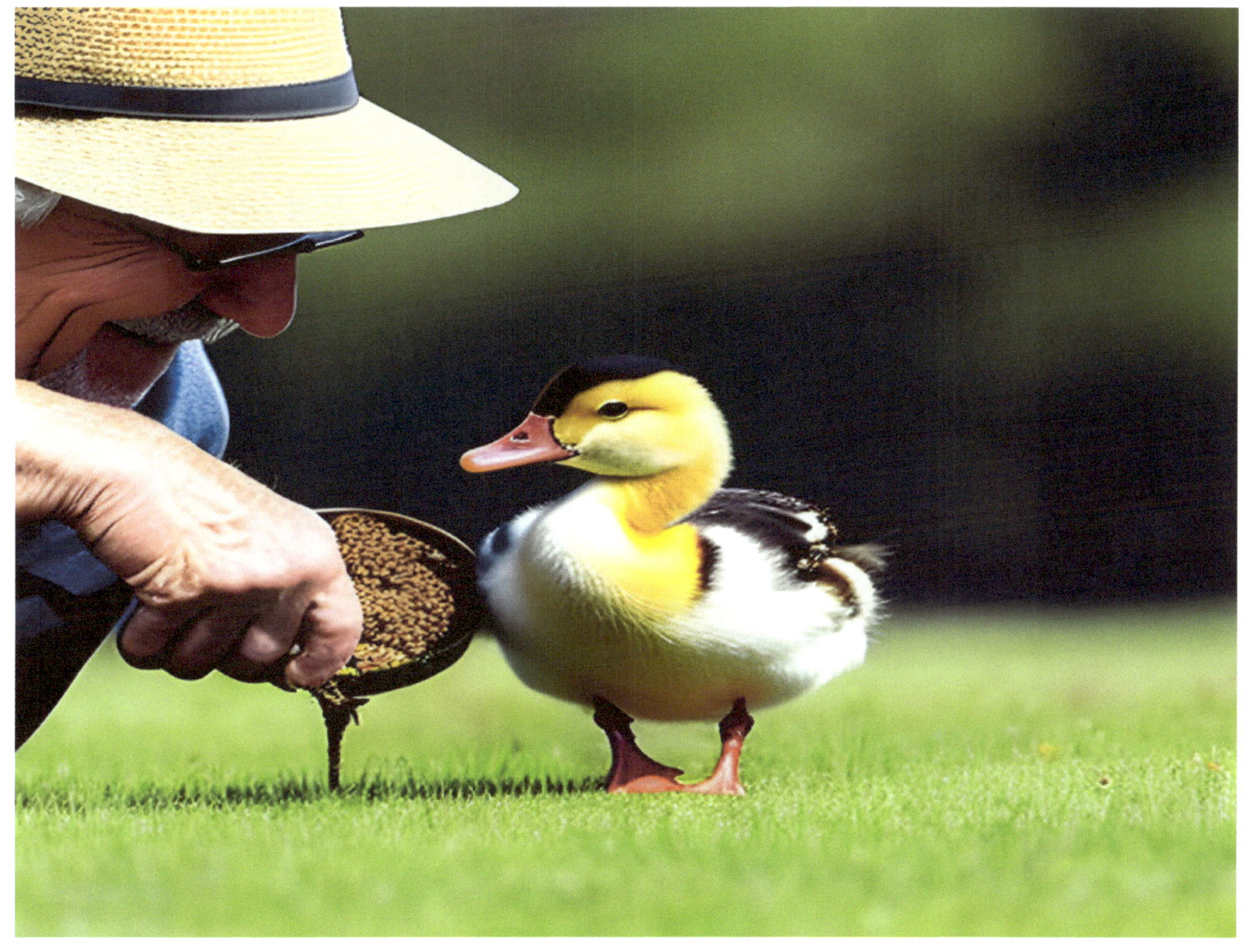

The farmer was so happy that Grace's dream finally came true, and he took special care of the two of them. He knew ducks ate a different diet than chickens, so he fed the chickens and then fed Frances her own special duck food in the hen house.

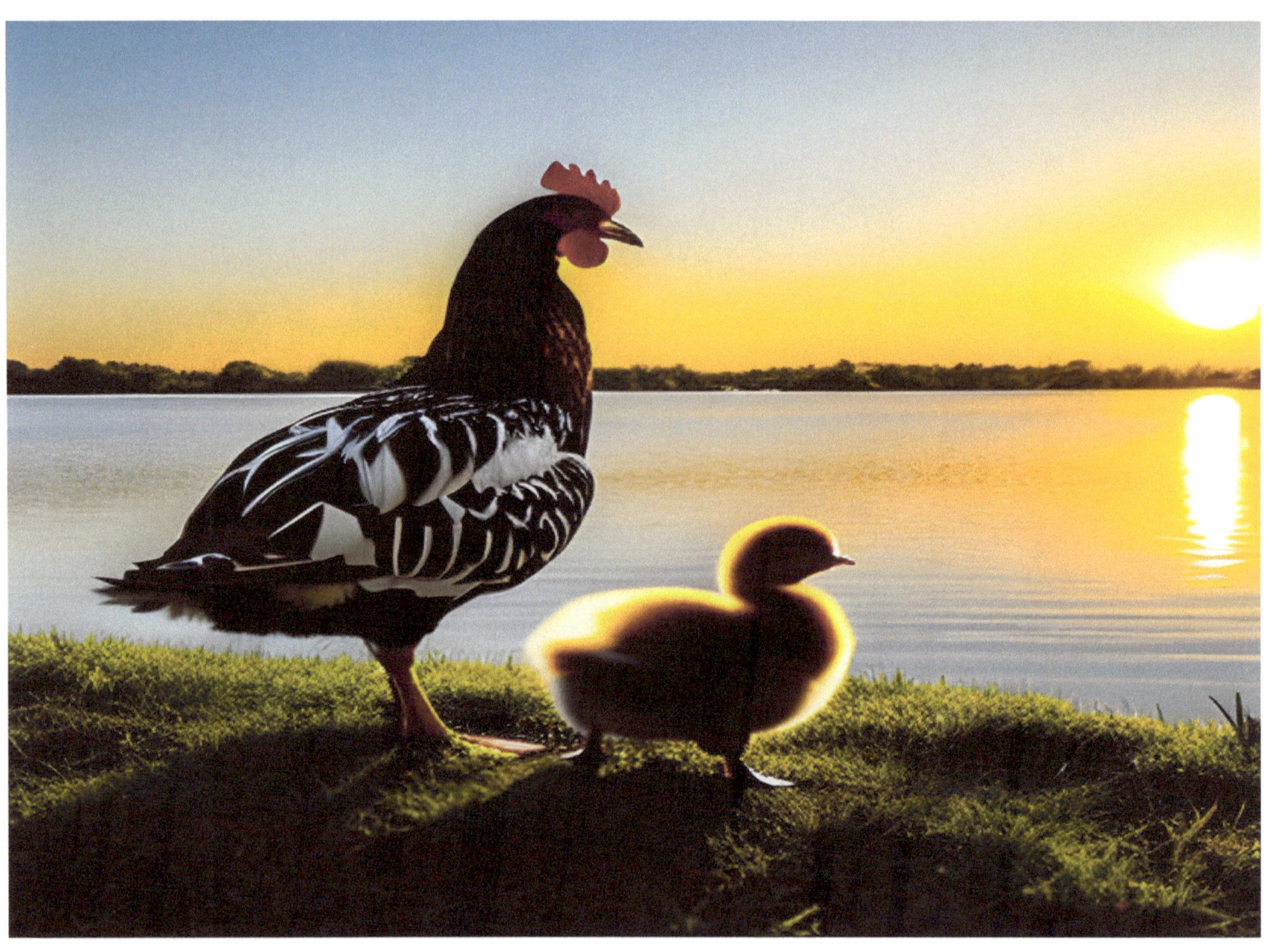

Grace and Frances lived a long happy life together and thankfully never had to endure another hurricane.

The End